Notice

Medicine is an ever-changing science. As new research and clinical experience broaden our knowledge, changes in treatment and drug therapy are required. The authors and the publisher of this work have checked with sources believed to be reliable in their efforts to provide information that is complete and generally in accord with the standards accepted at the time of publication. However, in view of the possibility of human error or changes in medical sciences, neither the authors nor the publisher nor any other party who has been involved in the preparation or publication of this work warrants that the information contained herein is in every respect accurate or complete, and they disclaim all responsibility for any errors or omissions or for the results obtained from use of the information contained in this work. Readers are encouraged to confirm the information contained herein with other sources. For example and in particular, readers are advised to check the product information sheet included in the package of each drug they plan to administer to be certain that the information contained in this work is accurate and that changes have not been made in the recommended dose or in the contraindications for administration. This recommendation is of particular importance in connection with new or infrequently used drugs.

a–z Common Symptom Answer Guide

John Wasson, MD
Herman O. West Chair of Geriatrics
Professor of Community and Family Medicine and Medicine
Dartmouth–Hitchcock Medical Center
Hanover, New Hampshire

Timothy Walsh, MD
Columbia University
College of Physicians & Surgeons
New York, New York

Mary C. LaBrecque, ARNP/MSN
Instructor in Community and Family Medicine
Dartmouth–Hitchcock Medical Center
Hanover, New Hampshire

Robert Pantell, MD
Professor of Pediatrics
University of California, San Francisco
San Francisco, California

Harold C. Sox, Jr., MD
Editor
Annals of Internal Medicine
Philadelphia, Pennsylvania

Ivan Oransky, MD
New York, New York

McGraw-Hill
MEDICAL PUBLISHING DIVISION

New York / Chicago / San Francisco / Lisbon / London
Madrid / Mexico City / Milan / New Delhi / San Juan
Seoul / Singapore / Sydney / Toronto

a–z Common Symptom Answer Guide

1 2 3 4 5 6 7 8 9 0   DOC/DOC   0 9 8 7 6 5 4

ISBN   0-07-141618-8

This book was set in New Aster by McGraw-Hill Professional's
Hightstown, NJ, composition unit.
The editor was Andrea Seils.
The production supervisor was Richard Ruzycka.
Project management was provided by Andover Publishing Services.
RR Donnelley was printer and binder.
This book was printed on acid-free paper.

Library of Congress Cataloging-in-Publication data is on file for this title at the Library of Congress.

Contents

When Something Feels Wrong

Symptoms are what you feel when your body's machinery isn't working perfectly. About twenty symptoms account for most of the reasons people go to health professionals. People visit a health professional when the symptoms limit daily activities. They also visit health professionals to learn whether their symptoms indicate an increased risk for serious problems.

The most common group of symptoms is caused when a "bug" (bacteria or virus) has invaded the body. The typical symptoms of a "bug" are cough, fever, chills, runny nose, sneezing, sore throat, earache, nausea, vomiting, and diarrhea. When caused by a "bug," these symptoms usually resolve within three weeks.

Symptoms caused by bacteria or viruses are particularly common in young children because the child's body is just learning how to fight the most common "bugs." We call this building up immunity. Immunizations are given to young children to help speed up this process and eliminate the problems caused when these bugs are able to invade the body. It's important to note that in children and adults, symptoms caused by viruses will not be helped by antibiotics.

The next most common symptoms are those related to "wear and tear" on the body. Low back, knee, leg, foot, hand, neck, and shoulder pains are most often caused by "wear and tear." These symptoms persist for weeks, months, or a lifetime.

After these two groupings, there a number of common symptoms with several or less obvious causes: headaches, abdominal (belly) pains, shortness of breath (difficulty breathing), chest pains, red or itching skin, emotional problems, dizziness, tiredness, and fatigue. These symptoms tend to occur again and again.

When Symptoms Limit Daily Activities

The more numerous, severe, and persistent our symptoms, the more they limit our ability to perform daily activities. Among adults, persistent "wear and tear" pains, anxiety or depression, dizziness or fatigue, and trouble sleeping frequently limit activities.

There are notable differences in the frequency of several bothersome, persistent symptoms by age and gender. Preteen, teen, and young women are more often bothered by headaches than males. Trouble paying attention is the most common problem for preteen and teen males. Sleep problems are more common as we age. Older people are frequently bothered by problems with urination, constipation, and hearing.

When Symptoms Might Indicate a Serious Problem

The overwhelming majority of symptoms are not a sign of a serious problem. That means that the body could heal itself without professional help. But large studies of symptoms show three interesting patterns.

First, while in children and adolescents the "bug-related" symptoms listed above are self-limited almost all of the time, fever and cough in the very old had a potentially serious cause about 5 to 10 times out of 100. The most common serious cause in the studies was an infection of the lung (pneumonia) that might have benefitted from antibiotics.

Second, about 5 to 10 out of 100 abdominal and chest pains suffered by adults in the studies were likely to have serious causes; in adolescents and children, these problems were very seldom serious.

Third, across all ages, shortness of breath (difficulty breathing) seemed to be the most common treatable symptom. About half of the time, professional treatment really helps cure or make less bothersome the causes for shortness of breath.

Symptoms Are Like Street Signs

What do these general patterns mean? If you are an older adult you should worry a bit more about cough, fever, chest pain, and abdominal pain. If you have persistent trouble breathing, see a health professional.

Unfortunately, a symptom is often just like a street sign. It can tell you roughly were you are, but without a specific address, you can easily end up in the wrong neighborhood. Cough is a common street sign for heart and lung problems. Cough with a fever of 103 degrees and shortness of breath that has lasted two days is closer to being an address for infection of the lung (pneumonia).

Combining such street signs, the way you would specify an address by providing the intersection of two streets, can help your doctor zoom in on a diagnosis. There's also common sense: Over millions of years, humans have survived because they "sense" when they are really sick. For example, rapidly progressive, severe symptoms usually require prompt action.

The *a–z Common Symptom Answer Guide* is intended to help you determine the possible causes for your symptoms, and to prepare you for what your doctor's visit for those symptoms may be like. It provides you with more than street signs—it places you in the correct neighborhood. But it won't establish a specific address or diagnosis. For example, the lungs need to be examined by a health professional to make the diagnosis and prescribe treatment for pneumonia. The *a–z Common Symptom Answer Guide* is not an adequate substitute for the judgment of a health professional—it's just a very helpful guide map.

John Wasson, MD

How to Use This Book

Feeling sick is, it goes without saying, a miserable experience. But on top of the aches, pains, and fatigue that go with many illnesses, there's the anxiety of not knowing what condition you might have, and not knowing what to expect when you go to your doctor's office.

There are many health resources available today, particularly on the Internet. Many, however, are meant for health care professionals, and among those that aren't, only a small percentage are accurate, with information vetted by doctors and nurses.

That's where the *a–z Common Symptom Answer Guide* comes in. Written in plain English —not the medicalese of *ER* or scientific journals—this book is designed to help you think about your symptoms and to prepare you for your doctor's visit. It can then be used as a handy reference after that visit to further explain and clarify anything you didn't have time to ask in the office or hospital.

The purpose is not to allow for self-diagnosis. Figuring out what ails you is for your doctor to do. But by knowing what questions your doctor might ask, you'll help her make a more definitive diagnosis. And by knowing what to expect, you'll hopefully rest easier and be more ready to cope with the information.

Organization

The book consists of seventy-five chapters, each named for a common symptom, instead of being organized by diseases or conditions. All the chapters are cross-referenced. That way, you can find the symptom you're experiencing, read about it, and, when appropriate, be referred to another chapter of related conditions. For an overview of terms or associations, refer to the Table of Contents, which lists all the chapters, and the Glossary, which defines common medical terms so you'll know what they mean when your doctor uses them. Different people have different names for symptoms and conditions; this way you'll be on the same page.

Each chapter begins with a "What it feels like" and "What can make it worse" section. Here, you'll find quick versions of what you might be experiencing. For example, certain medications can worsen some symptoms.

The next section of each chapter is "Your Doctor Visit." In that section, you'll find a list of questions your doctor might ask and a description of the examinations or tests he might perform. Many times, doctors can be guided quickly to the correct diagnosis by knowing the medical history of a patient or her family, but this information isn't always easily available. It's particularly easy to forget such details when you're not feeling well. If, before going to the doctor, you read through the questions you may be asked, you may avoid this problem.

The last section of each chapter is a table or list of conditions and diseases that might be causing your symptoms. Each condition is defined and described in clear English, with particular attention paid to what might distinguish a particular diagnosis from another. For example, many diseases can cause abdominal pain, but the exact location of your pain may tell you the difference between an ulcer, an inflamed appendix, or just constipation. The causes are ranked in order of common to rare when possible.

An important note: Read the "typical symptoms" column carefully when looking at the possible diagnoses, and don't assume the worst. For example, lung tumor is listed as one cause of hiccoughs. However, unless you have an unrelenting cough, are coughing up blood, or have a history of smoking cigarettes, it's highly unlikely that your hiccoughs are caused by a lung tumor.

Many of the chapters include additional statements and tidbits that may be of particular importance. For example, there are steps to take immediately after a child swallows a poison that won't wait until a doctor's visit.

Staying Well—and Well-Informed

When you've returned from your doctor's office or the hospital, refer again to the *a–z Common Symptom Answer Guide*. You may find it particularly helpful to look up conditions or terms that your doctor used, to remind yourself of what they mean. As your treatment progresses and your condition improves, you may also want to compare your symptoms to what they were before, and reading the chapters that describe them again may help.

It is also important to take an active role in your health, not just by reacting to symptoms when they arise but by living a healthy lifestyle that includes exercise. You can keep up with changes in your life or in medicine that may affect your health in many ways. Having a regular physical is one such way. Your doctor may recommend other material for your review and reference.

Be well!

Ivan Oransky, MD

Acknowledgments

I would like to thank Alison McCook for her invaluable help in writing this book. My father, Stanley Oransky, MD, also has my gratitude for offering advice and recommendations on the material covered. The patients, professors, editors, and colleagues who taught me about medicine and how to write deserve anonymous but generous appreciation. Finally, the book would not have been possible without the patience and talent of its editor, Andrea Seils, and the encouragement of Jack Farrell, both of McGraw-Hill.

Ivan Oransky, MD

a–z *Common Symptom Answer Guide*

Abdominal Pain (Adult)

What it feels like: varies from a gnawing pain near the top of your abdomen, to cramping pain in your lower abdomen, to sharp shooting pains in many areas.

What can make it worse: food, medications, alcohol, movement, position, bowel movements, emotional stress, menstruation.

What can make it better: food or milk, antacids, medications, position, bowel movements, passing gas, burping.

Your Doctor Visit

What your doctor will ask you about: changes in appetite or bowel habits, weight loss, fever, chills, chest pain, back pain, trouble breathing, cough, previous injury to the chest or abdomen, burning on urination, blood in your stool or urine, vomiting, diarrhea, constipation, relation of pain to menstrual cycle, vaginal discharge, the possibility of pregnancy, abnormal vaginal bleeding, vaginal pain.

Your doctor will want to know if you or anyone in your family has had any of these conditions: diabetes, heart disease, atrial fibrillation, abdominal surgery, appendicitis, kidney stones, gallbladder disease, hernia, ulcer, liver disease, Crohn's disease, ulcerative colitis.

Your doctor will want to know if you drink alcohol, and how much.

Your doctor will want to know if you're taking any of these medications: aspirin, other anti-inflammatory medications such as ibuprofen or naproxen, beta-blockers.

Your doctor will do a physical examination including the following: temperature, blood pressure, pulse, weight, listening to your chest with a stethoscope, pushing on your abdomen, listening

1

to your abdomen with a stethoscope, digital rectal examination (including testing your stool for blood), pelvic examination, thorough skin examination, tests of your hip joint for pain.

Your doctor may do the following blood tests: blood count, blood chemistry, liver function tests.

WHAT CAN CAUSE ABDOMINAL PAIN, AND WHAT IS TYPICAL FOR EACH CAUSE?

CAUSE	WHAT IS IT?	TYPICAL SYMPTOMS
Gastroenteritis	Infection of the stomach or intestines	Nausea, vomiting, diarrhea, cramping, muscle aches, slight fever
Heartburn	Also known as GERD (GastroEsophageal Reflux Disease), the movement of stomach acid up into and through the esophagus, which connects the throat to the stomach; can lead to ulcer (see below)	Burning upper abdominal pain, worse when lying flat or bending over, particularly soon after meals, relieved by antacids or sitting upright
Irritable bowel syndrome	Alternating diarrhea and constipation, sometimes occurring during periods of anxiety	Cramping, diarrhea, constipation, with minimal pain, no fever
Ulcer	Severe irritation of the stomach or intestinal lining	Burning upper abdominal pain that is worse when lying down, sometimes relieved by antacids and made worse by aspirin or drugs such as ibuprofen
Appendicitis	Infection or inflammation of the appendix, a small pouch of the large intestine	Pain in the lower right part of the abdomen, low-grade fever (less than 101 degrees F)
Hepatitis	Infection or inflammation of the liver, can be caused by viruses or by heavy long-term drinking	Weakness, fatigue, right upper abdominal pain, jaundice (skin taking on a yellowish appearance)

	WHAT CAN CAUSE ABDOMINAL PAIN, AND WHAT IS TYPICAL FOR EACH CAUSE? (CONTINUED)	
CAUSE	WHAT IS IT?	TYPICAL SYMPTOMS
Diverticulitis	Infection of pockets of the large intestine	Fever, pain in lower left part of the abdomen, constipation, nausea, vomiting, sometimes blood in the stool
Cholecystitis	Gallstones	Fever, right upper abdominal pain, sometimes pain in right shoulder, nausea, vomiting, chills, sometimes jaundice (skin taking on a yellowish appearance), dark urine
Pancreatitis	Inflammation of the pancreas, the organ that produces insulin, the glucose-regulating hormone, often associated with history of heavy drinking or gallstones	Pain in the upper abdomen, sometimes in the back, nausea, vomiting, sometimes weakness and rapid heart rate
Ureteral stone	Passing of a kidney stone into one of the ureters, the tubes that connect the kidney to the bladder	Pain usually begins in side, accompanied by painful urination and blood in the urine, can lead to fever
Ectopic pregnancy (in women)	Presence of a growing fetus outside the uterus, usually in the fallopian tubes	Missed menstrual period, severe lower abdominal pain that appears suddenly
Pelvic inflammatory disease (in women)	Inflammation of the reproductive tract that results from past sexually transmitted diseases	Severe pain in the lower abdomen, fever, chills, vaginal discharge, painful sexual intercourse
Ulcerative colitis	Inflammation of the rectum and colon	Low-grade fever (less than 101 degrees F), some pain in lower abdomen, blood may appear in stools, which are small and not well-formed, sometimes weight loss

WHAT CAN CAUSE ABDOMINAL PAIN, AND WHAT IS TYPICAL FOR EACH CAUSE? (CONTINUED)		
CAUSE	WHAT IS IT?	TYPICAL SYMPTOMS
Crohn's disease	Inflammation of the entire gastrointestinal system (can occur from mouth to rectum)	Low-grade fever (less than 101 degrees F), pain in lower right part of the abdomen that is often relieved by defecation of stools that are soft and not well-formed
Abdominal aortic aneurysm rupture	A tear of the aorta, the largest blood vessel in the body	Acute pain anywhere between the chest and lower abdomen, weakness, rapid heartbeat, sometimes a pulsing mass can be felt
Bowel infarction	Failure of blood to get to part of the intestine, leading to death of part of the intestine, often associated with a history of abdominal surgery	Weakness, rapid heartbeat, paleness, and sweating, distended belly, pain is all over abdomen
Peritonitis	An infection of the lining of the abdomen	Severe pain that worsens with movement, fever, rigidity
Bowel obstruction	A blockage in the intestines	Nausea, vomiting, sometimes constipation, distended belly, extreme discomfort
Heart attack	Blockage in one of the arteries feeding the heart, leading to death of part of the heart muscle	Pain is very severe in the chest or very high in the abdomen, possibly in the jaw or left shoulder and elbow, sweating

Abdominal Pain (Child)

What it feels like: varies from a gnawing pain near the top of your abdomen, to cramping pain in your lower abdomen, to sharp shooting pains in many areas.

What can make it worse: food, medications, movement, position, bowel movements, emotional stress.

What can make it better: food or milk, antacids, medications, position, bowel movements, passing gas, burping.

Your Doctor Visit

What your doctor will ask you and your child about: headache, coughing, vomiting, changes in bowel habits, the color of the stool, weight loss, constipation, blood or worms in stool, flank pain, blood in the urine, painful urination, joint pains, attention-seeking behavior.

Your doctor will want to know if your child or anyone in your family has had any of these conditions: recent "stomach bug," sickle-cell disease, mumps, or strep throat.

Your doctor will want to know whether your home has lead-based paint, and if you've seen your child eating paint chips.

Your doctor will want to know if your child is taking any medications.

Your doctor will do a physical examination including the following: temperature, blood pressure, pulse, weight, listening to your child's chest with a stethoscope, pushing on your child's abdomen, listening to your child's abdomen with a stethoscope, testing your child's stool for blood, thorough skin examination, tests of your child's hip joint for pain.

Your doctor may do the following blood tests: blood count, blood chemistry, liver function tests.

WHAT CAN CAUSE ABDOMINAL PAIN, AND WHAT IS TYPICAL FOR EACH CAUSE?		
CAUSE	**WHAT IS IT?**	**TYPICAL SYMPTOMS**
Gastroenteritis	Infection of the stomach or intestines	Nausea, vomiting, diarrhea, cramping, muscle aches, slight fever
Unclear cause	Alternating diarrhea and constipation, sometimes occurring during periods of anxiety	Attention-seeking behavior, cramping, diarrhea, constipation, with minimal pain, no fever
Colic	Crying spells seen between the ages of 2 weeks and 4 months, probably due to abdominal pain	Crying spells, usually resolves on its own by age of 4 months
Constipation	Constipation	Diffuse pain
Appendicitis (unlikely before the age of 3 years)	Infection or inflammation of the appendix, a small pouch of the large intestine	Pain in the lower right part of the abdomen, low-grade fever (less than 101 degrees F)
Pharyngitis	Sore throat, can lead to abdominal pain	Fever, enlarged "glands," sore throat, redness in throat
Pneumonia	Lung infection, can lead to abdominal pain because of coughing	Fever, cough
Mumps	Infection that causes the area around the cheeks to swell, now prevented in large part by vaccination (MMR = measles, *mumps*, rubella)	Swollen cheeks, fever
Lactose intolerance	Reaction to lactose, a sugar found in milk and cheese	Bloating, cramping pain

WHAT CAN CAUSE ABDOMINAL PAIN, AND WHAT IS TYPICAL FOR EACH CAUSE? (CONTINUED)

CAUSE	WHAT IS IT?	TYPICAL SYMPTOMS
Sickle-cell disease	Painful "crises" caused by misshapen red blood cells, an inherited disease found most often in African Americans	Severe pain in abdomen and joints, sweating, sometimes fever
Worms	Infection by *Ascaris*, hookworm, *Taenia*, *Strongyloides* species	Worms and eggs in stool, mild pain, weight loss, diarrhea
Lead poisoning	Caused by exposure to lead, most often in lead paint in older houses	Diffuse abdominal pain, can in the long term lead to mental retardation
Bowel obstruction	A blockage in the intestines	Nausea, vomiting, sometimes constipation, distended belly, extreme discomfort
Intussusception (common between ages of 5 months and 2 years)	"Telescoping" of tubes of intestines into one another	Slight fever, acute sudden pain, vomiting, often decreased bowel movements
Ulcer	Severe irritation of the stomach or intestinal lining	Burning upper abdominal pain that is worse when lying down, sometimes relieved by antacids and made worse by aspirin or ibuprofen
Henoch-Schönlein purpura	Inflammation of the blood vessels that often follows respiratory infections	Joint pain, vomiting, distended belly, bruising (occurs later)
Kidney disease	Congenital kidney problems (several)	Severity of pain varies, but generally over the flank
Hepatitis (unlikely)	Infection or inflammation of the liver, can be caused by viruses	Weakness, fatigue, right upper abdominal pain, jaundice (skin taking on a yellowish appearance)

WHAT CAN CAUSE ABDOMINAL PAIN, AND WHAT IS TYPICAL FOR EACH CAUSE? (CONTINUED)		
CAUSE	**WHAT IS IT?**	**TYPICAL SYMPTOMS**
Cholecystitis (unlikely in children)	Gallstones	Fever, right upper abdominal pain, sometimes pain in right shoulder, nausea, vomiting, chills, sometimes jaundice (skin taking on a yellowish appearance), dark urine
Pancreatitis (unlikely in children)	Inflammation of the pancreas, the organ that produces insulin, the glucose-regulating hormone, often associated with gallstones	Pain in the upper abdomen, sometimes in the back, nausea, vomiting, sometimes weakness and rapid heart rate
Ulcerative colitis (unlikely in children)	Inflammation of the rectum and colon	Low-grade fever (less than 101 degrees F), some pain in lower abdomen, blood may appear in stools, which are small and not well-formed, sometimes weight loss
Crohn's disease (unlikely in children)	Inflammation of the entire gastrointestinal system (can occur from mouth to rectum)	Low-grade fever (less than 101 degrees F), pain in lower right part of the abdomen that is often relieved by defecation of stools that are soft and not well formed

Allergic Symptoms (Sneezing, Runny Nose, or Hives)

What it feels like: varies from person to person, and includes a number of symptoms such as sniffling, sneezing, watery eyes, rash or other skin problems, which typically appear when you come in contact with a particular substance or animal, or during particular seasons.

This chapter describes what happens when you have allergies. However, some of these symptoms—such as sneezing and sniffling—also occur when you have a cold. Refer to chapters on Breathing Problems (Child), Cough, and Fever for more details.

Your Doctor Visit

What your doctor will ask you about: rash, hives, your reactions to insect bites, wheezing, difficulty breathing, your work, where you live, and whether you are exposed to dust, chemicals, or animals. Your doctor will also want to know whether you have ever been treated for allergies or asthma, or had skin testing for specific allergies performed.

Your doctor will ask if certain seasons, substances or animals "trigger" your symptoms, and if you feel better once those triggers disappear.

Your doctor will want to know if you or anyone in your family has had any of these conditions: drug allergies, asthma, eczema, hives, hay fever, food allergies.

Your doctor will want to know if you're taking any of these medications: steroids, bronchodilators, antihistamines, skin creams, allergy shots, decongestants.

Your doctor will do a physical examination including the following: pulse, blood pressure, eye exam, nose exam, listening to your chest with a stethoscope, thorough skin examination.

WHAT ARE SOME CONDITIONS THAT RESULT FROM ALLERGIES, AND WHAT IS TYPICAL FOR EACH CONDITION?		
CONDITION	**WHAT IS IT?**	**TYPICAL SYMPTOMS**
Rhinitis	Inflammation in the nose	Sneezing, runny and stuffy nose, watery eyes, post-nasal drip
Asthma	Severe breathing problem	Wheezing, difficulty breathing, chest constriction
Hives	Type of rash, generally bumpy or raised	Swelling on the skin that can itch or burn
Eczema	Type of scaly red rash	Redness on the skin that can ooze or become scaly and crusted
Anaphylaxis	Body-wide allergic reaction	Swelling of neck and face, trouble breathing, confusion, light-headedness, nausea, rash

Anus Problems

What it feels like: varies from itching, burning, or bleeding to pain, sometimes extreme.

What can make it worse: bowel movements, anal sex.

Your Doctor Visit

What your doctor will ask you about: pain, bleeding, burning, itching, swelling, discharge, constipation, diarrhea, loss of control of bowels, the presence of worms in stool, changes in urination. Your doctor will also want to know if another doctor has ever performed an anal or rectal examination on you, including with a special camera called a sigmoidoscope.

Your doctor will want to know if you or anyone in your family has had any of these conditions: hemorrhoids, liver disease, Crohn's disease, surgery to the anus or rectum, diabetes, worm infestations.

Your doctor will want to know if you're taking any of these medications: rectal ointments, enemas, antibiotics.

Your doctor will do a physical examination including the following: testing your stool for blood, rectal exam to check for tears, holes, or hemorrhoids, possibly using a tool called an anoscope to look inside your anus.

WHAT CAN CAUSE ANUS PROBLEMS, AND WHAT IS TYPICAL FOR EACH CAUSE?

CAUSE	WHAT IS IT?	TYPICAL SYMPTOMS
Hemorrhoids	Swollen blood vessels in the anus or rectum	Pain, bleeding, possibly a mass of smooth, bluish tissue
Dermatitis	Skin inflammation near the anus, a result of infection or scratching	Itching, anal area may be red, moist, blistery, and crusty
Fissures or fistulae	Tears in the tissue lining the anus (fissures) or holes (fistulae)	Anal tenderness, pain with bowel movements, itching, burning, constipation, discharge
Proctalgia	Sharp pain in the rectum	Recurrent, intermittent pain in the rectum lasting at least 20 minutes
Perirectal abscess	Collection of pus as a result of an infection	Extreme throbbing pain
Prostatitis	Inflammation within the prostate	Changes in urination, lower abdominal pain
Intestinal parasite	Infection with organisms such as pinworms, hookworms, or tapeworms	Itching, worms in vomit or bowel movements, diarrhea, abdominal discomfort
Cancer	An abnormal growth of cells, may begin as a benign growth (polyp)	Blood in stools, changes in habits related to bowel movements

Back Pain

What it feels like: stiffness and pain centered anywhere in the back, sometimes radiating into the legs or buttocks, and possibly originating after heavy lifting or injury.

What can make it worse: coughing, sneezing, walking, movement, menstruation.

What can make it better: antacids, leaning forward, bed rest.

The most common form of back pain results from strain in the lower back.

Your Doctor Visit

What your doctor will ask you about: urinary incontinence, difficulty or pain with urinating, blood in urine, pain or numbness in the buttocks or legs, abdominal pain, hip pain, fever or chills, nausea, vomiting, flank pain, vaginal discharge. Your doctor will also want to know whether you have ever had an X-ray, CT scan, or MRI of your spine, or any other tests of your backbone, and what they showed, and whether you have ever had surgery on your spine.

Your doctor will want to know if your back pain began after a back injury or fall, and the precise location of the pain.

Your doctor will want to know if you or anyone in your family has had any of these conditions: cancer, recent surgery, spinal fracture.

Your doctor will want to know if you're taking any regular medications, particularly steroids or anticoagulants.

Your doctor will do a physical examination including the following: pushing on your abdomen, listening to your abdomen with

13

a stethoscope, pelvic exam (in women), muscle spasms in the back, tenderness in the back, spinal curvature and flexibility, reflexes in the legs and feet, strength and sensation in the feet and calves.

WHAT CAN CAUSE BACK PAIN, AND WHAT IS TYPICAL FOR EACH CAUSE?		
CAUSE	**WHAT IS IT?**	**TYPICAL SYMPTOMS**
Muscle strain	Injury to muscles	Muscle spasms near the spine, pain does not move to the legs, often begins after lifting
Spinal fracture	A break in one of the bones of the spine, called vertebrae	Severe, persistent pain, tenderness, often the result of back injury or fall
Osteomyelitis	Bone infection	Constant and progressive back pain lasting several weeks, may be history of recent infection
Osteoarthritis	The most common form of arthritis, or inflammation of the joints	Limited range of motion of the spine, often accompanied by pain in other joints, more common in the elderly
Ankylosing spondylitis	Arthritis affecting the spine	Stiffness, lower back pain, reduced flexibility in the spine, more common in young men
Shingles	Re-activation of the virus that causes chicken pox; more common in the elderly who have had chicken pox	Painful skin sores
Peptic ulcer	Severe irritation of the stomach lining	Abdominal pain or tenderness, pain in the mid-back region, sometimes relieved by antacids

	WHAT CAN CAUSE BACK PAIN, AND WHAT IS TYPICAL FOR EACH CAUSE? (CONTINUED)	
CAUSE	**WHAT IS IT?**	**TYPICAL SYMPTOMS**
Pancreatitis	Inflammation of the pancreas, the organ that produces insulin, which regulates sugar; often associated with history of heavy drinking or gallstones	Pain in the upper abdomen, sometimes in the back, nausea, vomiting, sometimes weakness and rapid heart rate
Abdominal aortic aneurysm	A swelling in the aorta, the largest blood vessel in the body	Acute upper abdominal pain, sometimes a pulsing can be felt in abdomen, more common in people over 50
Kidney stones (See chapter on Urine Problems.)	The presence of a stone made up of mineral salts in the kidney	History of passing blood or "gravel" in urine, severe pain radiating to groin or testicle
Pyelonephritis	Kidney infection	Pain in the sides, upper abdominal tenderness, difficulty or pain with urination, blood in urine, fever
Gynecologic disease	Disease affecting the reproductive organs in women	Pain in the lower part of the abdomen or sacrum, vaginal discharge, pain may change according to menstruation
Prostatitis	Infection or inflammation of prostate	Changes in urination, lower abdominal pain
Neurological damage	Damage to the spinal cord	Pain radiating to legs, inability to move legs, trouble moving legs, bladder problems, often the result of spinal fracture (see page 14) caused by an injury
Herniated intervertebral disk	A disk between vertebrae protrudes into the space that holds the spinal cord, squeezing it	Pain radiating into legs or buttocks, aggravated by sneezing or coughing, often begins after lifting

WHAT CAN CAUSE BACK PAIN, AND WHAT IS TYPICAL FOR EACH CAUSE? (CONTINUED)		
CAUSE	WHAT IS IT?	TYPICAL SYMPTOMS
Spinal stenosis	A narrowing of the spinal column that leads to a pinching of the spinal cord and nerves	Unsteady walk, thigh weakness, lower back pain that radiates into the thighs, often relieved by bending forward
Tumor in vertebrae	Malignant and abnormal growth of cells in the vertebrae, the bones that make up the spine	Severe, progressive pain, more common in older patients and people with a history of cancer

Bed Wetting (Child)

Many factors can trigger a child's tendency to wet the bed, a behavior seen in up to one-fifth of children under the age of 10. Most children who wet the bed do not have "accidents" during the day.

Your Doctor Visit

What your doctor will ask you about: how often the child wets the bed, if she has "accidents" during the day, if she is excessively hungry or thirsty, if she produces a large amount of urine or has trouble or pain with urination, seizures, numbness, or weakness, emotional or disciplinary problems, sleeping habits.

Your doctor will want to know if the child or anyone in her family has had any of these conditions: diabetes, seizures, kidney diseases, bed wetting.

Your doctor may ask about the child's home environment, such as the birth of a new sibling or other recent changes, and how the child was toilet-trained.

Your doctor will do a physical examination including the following: pushing on the child's abdomen, thorough examination of strength, reflexes, and sensation, tests of the child's developmental skills.

WHAT CAN CAUSE BED WETTING IN CHILDREN, AND WHAT IS TYPICAL FOR EACH CAUSE?		
CAUSE	WHAT IS IT?	TYPICAL SYMPTOMS
Psychological	Stress or other emotional problems, such as difficulty reacting to the birth of a new sibling or other changes, often in children whose families have histories of bed wetting	No "accidents" during the day
Diabetes or kidney disease	These conditions can damage the kidneys	Excessive thirst, producing a large amount of urine, dribbling urine, or having difficulty or pain with urination
Seizures	Convulsions	Seizures that occur prior to bed wetting
Neurologic disease	Abnormalities in the nervous system	Bed wetting is associated with neurological problems such as mental retardation

Blackouts

What it feels like: temporarily losing consciousness or vision, some-times preceded by feeling faint or giddy.

What can make it worse: coughing, urination, head-turning, exer-tion, pain, a fright, food, hitting your head.

Your Doctor Visit

What your doctor will ask you about: seizures, changes in vision, changes in sensation or movement, urination and bowel movements, chest pain, hunger, sweating, dizziness when standing, head injuries.

Your doctor will want to know if you or anyone in your family has had any of these conditions: seizures, neurologic disease, dia-betes, cardiovascular disease, lung disease.

Your doctor will want to know what happened when you blacked out, including what position you were in, and whether anyone watched you black out.

Your doctor will want to know if you're taking any of these med-ications: digitalis, antiarrhythmics, anticonvulsants, antidepres-sants, blood pressure medications, insulin, diuretics, oral hypo-glycemic agents.

Your doctor will do a physical examination including the fol-lowing: blood pressure, pulse, listening to your heart with a stethoscope, testing your stool for blood, thorough neurological examination.

WHAT CAN CAUSE BLACKOUTS, AND WHAT IS TYPICAL FOR EACH CAUSE?		
CAUSE	**WHAT IS IT?**	**TYPICAL SYMPTOMS**
Vasovagal/ postural syncope	Common fainting	Blacking out after standing, coughing, urinating, emotional stress, or injury
Insufficient cardiac output	Your heart is not pumping enough blood to meet your body's needs	History of heart disease, chest pain, or irregular heart beats, blackouts may occur after exercise
Cerebrovascular disease	Blockages of the blood vessels feeding the brain	Spontaneous falls, sometimes changes in vision, speech, or movement
Seizures (See chapter on Convulsions [Seizures].)	Convulsions	Losing control of your movements, an alternating pattern of rigidity and relaxation, sometimes accompanied by a loss of consciousness; sometimes accompanied by loss of bowel or bladder control
Anemia (See chapter on Weakness.)	Low blood count	Black bowel movements, rapid heart rate
Medication use	Diuretics, blood pressure medications, antidepressants, digitalis, insulin	Hunger, sweating, heart pounding prior to losing consciousness, fainting after standing
Psychological	Stress or other emotional problems	Prolonged "coma" without any clear cause, may feature eyelid fluttering

Bloating

What it feels like: swelling and/or discomfort in the belly that occurs after eating.

What can make it worse: meals, certain positions, eating particular foods.

What can make it better: antacids, belching.

If you also feel abdominal pain, refer to the chapter on that subject for more information.

Your Doctor Visit

What your doctor will ask you about: abdominal pain, nausea, vomiting, change in bowel habits, black stools, change in abdominal girth, greasy bowel movements, weight change, gas, belching, regurgitation, anxiety, depression, relation of bloating to bowel movements, results of previous X-rays or ultrasound examinations.

Your doctor will want to know if you or anyone in your family has had any of these conditions: abdominal surgery, ulcer disease, colitis, diverticulosis, alcoholism, liver disease, hiatus hernia, obesity, emotional problems.

Your doctor will want to know the nature of your pain and where it occurs.

Your doctor will want to know if you're taking any of these medications: diuretics ("water pills"), heart medications such as calcium channel agents, antidepressants, tranquilizers, antacids, antispasmodics (Librax, belladonna).

Your doctor will do a physical examination including the following: weight, pushing on the abdomen, checking stool for the presence of blood.

WHAT CAN CAUSE BLOATING, AND WHAT IS TYPICAL FOR EACH CAUSE?		
CAUSE	WHAT IS IT?	TYPICAL SYMPTOMS
Aerophagia	Swallowing air	Bloating, belching, gas, chronic, worsened with certain foods
Flatulence	Passing gas	Bloating, belching, gas, chronic, worsened with certain foods
Digestion problems	Includes the inability to digest certain foods and difficulty absorbing nutrients from foods	Diarrhea caused by certain foods, greasy bowel movements, weight loss
Gastrointestinal problems (See chapter on Abdominal Pain.)	A disorder of the stomach or intestines	Weight loss, abdominal pain, change in bowel habits, nausea, vomiting
Ascites	Abnormal collection of fluid in the abdomen due to liver disease	Swollen belly, more common in people with a history of alcoholism and liver disease
Colic	Sudden and sharp abdominal pain	Brief episodes of crying and writhing, bowel sounds, often relieved by passing gas; occurs only in newborns and infants
Irritable bowel syndrome	Alternating diarrhea and constipation, sometimes occurring during periods of anxiety	Cramping, diarrhea, constipation, with minimal pain, no fever

Blood in Stool

What it looks like: a mixing of blood with bowel movements, making the toilet water red or streaking stool or toilet paper.

Eating certain things can change the color of your stool. For instance, beets can turn stool red, while iron pills and bismuth (Pepto-Bismol) can turn stool black.

Your Doctor Visit

What your doctor will ask you about: abdominal pain, changes in bowel habits or stool, mucus or pus in stool, pain with bowel movements, nausea, vomiting, heartburn, vomiting blood, bruising, weight loss, dizziness when standing, whether you have had a barium enema, proctoscope, or abdominal X-ray done in the past, and what they showed.

Your doctor will want to know if you or anyone in your family has had any of these conditions: hemorrhoids, diverticulosis, colitis, peptic ulcers, bleeding tendency, alcoholism, colon polyps.

Your doctor will want to know if you're taking any of these medications: warfarin (Coumadin), adrenal steroids, aspirin, anti-inflammatory drugs.

Your doctor will do a physical examination including the following: blood pressure, pulse, pushing on your abdomen, checking your rectum for hemorrhoids, testing your stool for blood, thorough skin examination.

**WHAT CAN CAUSE BLOOD IN STOOL,
AND WHAT IS TYPICAL FOR EACH CAUSE?**

IN ADULTS

CAUSE	WHAT IS IT?	TYPICAL SYMPTOMS
Hemorrhoids/ anal fissure (See chapter on Anus Problems.)	Swollen blood vessels in the anus or rectum (hemorrhoids) or tears in the tissue lining the anus (fissures)	Rectal pain, light bleeding
Angiodysplasia/ diverticular disease	Swollen, weakened blood vessels in the colon, leading to loss of blood	Bright red stool, minimal pain
Ulcer (See chapter on Abdominal Pain (Adult).)	Severe irritation of the stomach or intestinal lining	Black, tar-like bowel movements, vomiting, burning upper abdominal pain that is worse when lying down, sometimes relieved by food or antacids and made worse by aspirin or drugs such as ibuprofen
Ulcerative colitis	Inflammation of the colon and rectum	Low-grade fever (less than 101 degrees F), some pain in lower abdomen, blood may appear in stools, which are small and not well-formed, sometimes weight loss
Gastritis	Infection of the stomach	Black, tar-like bowel movements, vomiting, upper abdominal pain and tenderness
Esophageal varices	Swollen blood vessels in the esophagus	Black, tar-like bowel movements, vomiting, vomiting blood, jaundice (skin taking on a yellowish appearance), spiderweb-like collection of blood vessels near the skin surface
Intestinal tumors or polyps	An abnormal growth of cells, may begin as a benign growth (polyp)	Blood in stools, constipation, weight loss, pain

WHAT CAN CAUSE BLOOD IN STOOL, AND WHAT IS TYPICAL FOR EACH CAUSE? (CONTINUED)

IN INFANTS

CAUSE	WHAT IS IT?	TYPICAL SYMPTOMS
Swallowed blood	Occurs while breast-feeding or during delivery	Dark, tar-like stools
Hemorrhagic disease	Excess bleeding	Bruising, bright red blood, dark, tar-like stools

IN CHILDREN

CAUSE	WHAT IS IT?	TYPICAL SYMPTOMS
Fissures or polyps	Tears in the tissue lining the anus (fissures) or benign growths (polyps)	Red blood streaks in stool
Constipation (See chapter on Constipation (Child).)	Inability to have bowel movements	Bright red blood in stool
Meckel's diverticulum	Tiny pouch located on the wall of the lower bowel, a vestige from the umbilical cord and fetal intestines; rare	No pain
Volvulus or intussusception	Congenital shift in the position of the intestine, which sometimes leads to obstruction; rare	Vomiting, decrease in bowel movements, abdominal pain

Breast Problems

What it feels like: varies from pain, tenderness, enlargement, or lumps to discharge from the nipple.

What can make it worse: different phases of the menstrual cycle, nursing, trauma.

Your Doctor Visit

What your doctor will ask you about: enlargement, pain, discharge, lumps, change in skin color, excessive milk production, fever, chills, mammography, swelling or lumps in the armpit.

Your doctor will want to know if you or anyone in your family has had any of these conditions: pregnancy, tuberculosis, nervous system disease, breast cancer, benign cystic disease, alcoholism, liver disease.

Your doctor will want to know if you're taking any of these medications: oral contraceptives, digoxin, phenothiazines such as Haldol, spironolactone (Aldactone), diphenylhydantoin (Dilantin), cimetidine (Tagamet).

Your doctor will do a physical examination including the following: thorough breast exam, checking lymph nodes under your arms, and, in males, checking testes for size and firmness.

WHAT CAN CAUSE BREAST PROBLEMS, AND WHAT IS TYPICAL FOR EACH CAUSE?

BREAST ENLARGEMENT

CAUSE	WHAT IS IT?	TYPICAL SYMPTOMS
Puberty	Period of becoming sexually mature, or capable of reproducing	Enlargement of one or both breasts, common and normal in male and female adolescents
Long-term use of certain medications	Use of spironolactone (Aldactone), digoxin (Lanoxin), diphenyl-hydantoin (Dilantin), cimetidine (Tagamet)	Breast enlargement in adult men
Liver disease	Includes hepatitis and cirrhosis (scarring of the liver)	Breast enlargement in adult men, jaundice (skin taking on a yellowish appearance), alcoholism, small and soft testicles
Testicular cancer	An abnormal growth of cells in the testicles	Breast enlargement in adult men, firm mass in the testicles

LUMPS OR MASSES

CAUSE	WHAT IS IT?	TYPICAL SYMPTOMS
Cystic mastitis	Fluid-filled sacs in the breast	Lumps in the breast, usually becoming painful before each menstrual period
Cancer	An abnormal growth of cells in the breast	Family history of breast cancer, lump with an ill-defined border, sometimes with dimpling of the overlying skin

**WHAT CAN CAUSE BREAST PROBLEMS,
AND WHAT IS TYPICAL FOR EACH CAUSE? (CONTINUED)**

BREAST PAIN

CAUSE	WHAT IS IT?	TYPICAL SYMPTOMS
Hormonal engorgement	Swelling of breast tissue in response to hormonal changes	Pain or tenderness in early pregnancy or during certain phases of menstrual cycle, pain sometimes aggravated by oral contraceptives
Mastitis	Inflammation in the breast, often caused by an infection	Fever, tender and swollen breasts, discharge, more common among nursing women

NIPPLE DISCHARGE

CAUSE	WHAT IS IT?	TYPICAL SYMPTOMS
Cancer	An abnormal growth of cells in the breast	Itching, scaling, discharge (which may include blood), lumps in the breast and under the armpits; later in the disease, the skin may become affected
Phenothiazines	Use of drugs such as Haldol	Clear or white discharge from the nipples
Puberty	Part of normal development, in the early teens	Clear or white discharge from the nipples

Breathing Problems (Adult)

What it feels like: an inability to breathe in and out with ease, which can occur suddenly or develop over time, and may be accompanied by other symptoms, including chest pain, light-headedness, or cough.

What can make it worse: dust, chest injury, lying down, exertion, breathing in a particular substance, prolonged inactivity, recent surgery, certain times of year, allergies, emotional stress.

What can make it better: certain medications, sitting or standing upright.

Your Doctor Visit

What your doctor will ask you about: anxiety, confusion, light-headedness, lethargy, fever, chills, night sweats, blueness or numbness in lips or fingers, cough, coughing up sputum or blood, wheezing, noisy breathing, swelling, weight change, the influence of being upright on your ability to breathe, chest pain, ankle swelling, previous chest X-rays, electrocardiograms, tests of lung function, allergy skin tests.

Your doctor will want to know if you or anyone in your family has had any of these conditions: heart disease, high blood pressure, obesity, pneumonia, chest surgery, anemia, tuberculosis, AIDS, allergies to drugs, eczema, hay fever, lung failure, chronic lung diseases such as bronchitis, emphysema, or fibrosis.

Your doctor will want to know if you smoke cigarettes and, if so, how many and for how long.

Your doctor may also ask where you have lived and if you have worked in certain professions linked to breathing problems, such as mining, stone carving, painting, and quarry work.

Your doctor will want to know if you're taking any of these medications: medications for asthma, digitalis, diuretics ("water pills"), medications for high blood pressure, steroids, antihistamines, decongestants, allergy shots, antibiotics, inhalants, beta-blockers, oral contraceptives.

Your doctor will do a physical examination including the following: blood pressure, pulse, breathing rate, weight, temperature, listening to your chest and heart with a stethoscope, thorough neck exam, checking your arms and legs for swelling or discoloration, pushing on your abdomen, thorough skin exam. Your doctor will also do an electrocardiogram (EKG), depending on your symptoms.

WHAT CAN CAUSE BREATHING PROBLEMS IN ADULTS, AND WHAT IS TYPICAL FOR EACH CAUSE?		
CAUSE	**WHAT IS IT?**	**TYPICAL SYMPTOMS**
Asthma	Recurrent attacks of wheezing, coughing, and shortness of breath brought on by certain triggers	Attacks typically occur after exposure to certain triggers, such as pollen, respiratory infections, animals
Anemia (See chapter on Weakness.)	Low blood count	Easy fatigue, dizziness that occurs in certain positions, pallor, sometimes blood present in stool
Obesity	Excess body weight	Worsening symptoms with more weight gain, breathing troubles appear with exertion or bending, no history of heart or lung disease
Foreign body aspiration	Accidentally breathing in a foreign substance that blocks airways	Range from wheezing and rapid breathing to gasping, turning blue, and losing consciousness unless object is removed from throat; symptoms typically begin while eating
Hyperventilation	Rapid, deep breathing	Sudden onset, anxiety, chest pain, light-headedness, tingling in the arms, legs, and around the mouth

WHAT CAN CAUSE BREATHING PROBLEMS IN ADULTS, AND WHAT IS TYPICAL FOR EACH CAUSE? *(CONTINUED)*		
Cause	**What Is It?**	**Typical Symptoms**
Pneumonia	Lung infection	Coughing up green or yellow sputum, fever or shaking, chills, coughing up blood, chest pain, rapid breathing
Pneumothorax	"Collapsed lung": an abnormal collection of air between the lungs and chest wall	Sudden onset of breathing trouble, chest pain, may occur after chest injury
Congestive heart failure	Heart becomes unable to pump enough blood to meet the body's needs	Trouble breathing with exertion or at night, history of heart disease or high blood pressure, weight gain
Respiratory failure	A condition in which the lungs cannot completely get rid of carbon dioxide	Confusion, lethargy, sleepiness, shallow and rapid breathing
Pulmonary edema	A collection of fluid in the lungs	Severe breathing problems that worsen when lying down, rapid breathing, coughing up sputum
Chronic obstructive pulmonary disease (COPD)	Lung diseases in which the lungs become damaged and do not work properly	Cough, coughing up sputum, worsening after waking from sleep, more common in heavy smokers and people exposed to industrial dusts
Tuberculosis	Lung infection that can spread to other parts of the body	Fever, night sweats, weight loss, chronic cough, coughing up blood, most common in people with compromised immunity, such as people with AIDS
Pulmonary infarction or emboli	The obstruction of a blood vessel feeding the lungs (embolus), sometimes causing tissue death in the lungs (infarction)	Chest pain, apprehension, sweating, feeling faint, cough, coughing up blood, rapid breathing, sometimes history of calf pain or leg immobilization, such as on long trips

WHAT CAN CAUSE BREATHING PROBLEMS IN ADULTS, AND WHAT IS TYPICAL FOR EACH CAUSE? (CONTINUED)		
CAUSE	WHAT IS IT?	TYPICAL SYMPTOMS
Lung tumor	An abnormal growth of cells in the lung	Change in cough patterns, coughing up blood, chest ache, more common in cigarette smokers

Breathing Problems (Child)

What it feels like: an inability to breathe in and out with ease, which can occur suddenly or develop over time, and may be accompanied by other symptoms, such as wheezing or coughing.

What can make it worse: dust, injury, exertion, breathing in a certain substance, particular times of the year, allergies, stress.

Healthy infants can experience "rattling" or noisy breathing until up to 5 months of age, while their respiratory systems develop.

Your Doctor Visit

What your doctor will ask you about your child: anxiety, change in voice, drooling, sore throat, trouble swallowing, decreased eating, cough, coughing up sputum, wheezing, blueness of lips or fingers, fever, chills, weight loss, chest pain, ankle swelling, confusion, lethargy. The doctor will also want to know if there is a history of exposure to dust or whether the child has inhaled a foreign body, how long the breathing problem has gone on, and whether the child has ever had a chest X-ray, and if so, what it showed.

Your doctor will want to know if the child or anyone in the child's family has had any of these conditions: asthma, lung disease, heart disease, cystic fibrosis, pneumonia, tuberculosis, measles, other recent infectious diseases, allergies to drugs, eczema, hay fever, emphysema, respiratory failure.

Your doctor will want to know if the child is taking any medications, including: steroids, asthma medications, antihistamines, decongestants, allergy shots, antibiotics, inhalants, beta-blocking agents.

Your doctor will do a physical examination of the child, including the following: temperature, pulse, respiration rate, weight, checking throat for swollen tonsils and redness, thorough neck exam, checking for flaring nostrils, listening to the chest and heart with a stethoscope, thorough skin exam, checking arms and legs for swelling or blueness.

WHAT CAN CAUSE BREATHING PROBLEMS IN CHILDREN, AND WHAT IS TYPICAL FOR EACH CAUSE?		
CAUSE	WHAT IS IT?	TYPICAL SYMPTOMS
Asthma	Recurrent attacks of wheezing, coughing, and shortness of breath brought on by certain triggers	Attacks typically caused by exposure to certain triggers, nighttime cough
Bronchiolitis	Infection of some of the tiny branches of the lungs	Fever, rapid breathing, wheezing, flaring nostrils, more common in infants less than 6 months old
Croup	Infection in the voicebox	Barking cough, wheezing, fever, hoarseness, typically appears after a cold, more common in children between 6 months and 3 years old
Epiglottitis	Infection or inflammation of the flap in the back of the throat that blocks air passages during swallowing	Vibrating sound during breathing, muffled speaking, sore throat, trouble swallowing, fever, drooling, most common in children between 3 and 7 years old
Hyperventilation	Rapid, shallow breathing	Sudden onset of breathing trouble, anxiety, chest pain (adolescents), light-headedness, tingling around the mouth, numbness in hands, more common in children older than 6 years
Pneumonia	Infection of the lungs	Coughing up sputum, high fever, rapid breathing

WHAT CAN CAUSE BREATHING PROBLEMS IN CHILDREN, AND WHAT IS TYPICAL FOR EACH CAUSE? (CONTINUED)		
CAUSE	WHAT IS IT?	TYPICAL SYMPTOMS
Pneumothorax	"Collapsed lung": an abnormal collection of air between the lungs and chest wall	Sudden onset, may occur after chest injury, more common in children with asthma
Chronic heart or respiratory disease	Long-term diseases that affect the heart or respiratory organs, such as cystic fibrosis or heart abnormalities	Less-than-average growth, attacks of shortness of breath, decreased feeding (in the newborn), consistent inability to exercise
Foreign body aspiration	Accidentally breathing in a foreign body that blocks airways	Range from wheezing and rapid breathing to gasping, turning blue, and losing consciousness, typically beginning with a gag, gasp, or cough

Breathing troubles in children can also be caused by lung collapse, fibrocystic disease, and chronic infections such as tuberculosis, producing symptoms that include cough, weight loss, recurrent lung infections, and coughing up sputum.

Bruising and Bleeding Tendencies

What it feels like: being quick to bruise after minor injury, spontaneous bleeding, or bleeding for long periods of time after a cut.

All bleeding disorders are characterized by a tendency to bruise easily.

Your Doctor Visit

What your doctor will ask you about: fever, chills, headache, swollen lymph nodes, joint swelling, dark or bloody urine, black and tar-like bowel movements, jaundice (skin taking on a yellowish appearance), skin rashes, infections.

Your doctor will want to know if you or anyone in your family has had any of these conditions: liver disease, valvular heart disease, hemophilia, systemic lupus erythematosus, tendency toward easy bruising or excess bleeding at the time of birth or later, particularly during surgeries or dental work.

Your doctor will want to know if you're taking any medications, including: steroids, diuretics ("water pills"), warfarin (Coumadin).

Your doctor will do a physical examination including the following: temperature, listening to your heart with a stethoscope, pushing on your abdomen, checking joints for swelling, thorough skin exam, checking lymph nodes to see if they are enlarged.

If you are going to have elective or nonelective surgery, be sure to tell your surgeon about your bruising or bleeding tendency.

WHAT CAN CAUSE A TENDENCY TO BRUISE OR BLEED EXCESSIVELY, AND WHAT IS TYPICAL FOR EACH CAUSE?		
CAUSE	**EXAMPLES**	**TYPICAL SYMPTOMS**
Lack or poor function of substances in the blood that enable it to clot	Hereditary disease (hemophilia), medication use (warfarin and other anticoagulants), liver disease	Large superficial bruises, spontaneous bleeding
Lack or poor function of blood particles called platelets, or fragile blood vessels	Medication use (diuretics and steroids), leukemia, diseases of the blood vessels, infections (bacterial infections of the heart, Rocky Mountain spotted fever)	Small, superficial bruises, prolonged bleeding, spot-sized bleeding into the skin

Burns

What it feels like: pain, blistering, and charred skin caused by injury from electricity, fire, or chemicals.

Your Doctor Visit

What your doctor will ask you about: pain, blistering, trouble breathing, loss of consciousness. If the burn was electrical, the doctor will ask where the source touched you, and what the source was.

Your doctor will want to know exactly where on your body you were burned, and the source of the burn. If it was a flame, the doctor will want to know if your face was burned. If the burn was chemical, the doctor will want to know what kind of chemical it was, whether there was contact to your face or eyes, and whether you swallowed any of it.

Your doctor will want to know when you had your last tetanus shot, and how many tetanus shots you have received in your life.

Your doctor will do a physical examination including the following: blood pressure, pulse, breathing rate, thorough skin exam.

WHAT ARE THE DIFFERENT TYPES OF BURNS, AND WHAT IS TYPICAL FOR EACH TYPE?		
BURN TYPE	**WHAT IS IT?**	**TYPICAL SYMPTOMS**
First-degree	Affects only the outermost layer of skin	Pain, red and dry skin, able to feel pinprick on burned skin
Second-degree	Affects outermost and an additional layer of skin	Mostly painful, blisters, underlying moist and red tissue, often able to feel pinprick on burned skin

WHAT ARE THE DIFFERENT TYPES OF BURNS, AND WHAT IS TYPICAL FOR EACH TYPE? (CONTINUED)		
BURN TYPE	**WHAT IS IT?**	**TYPICAL SYMPTOMS**
Third-degree	Burn affects deep tissues, beyond outermost layers	No pain, charred or leathery skin, skin may be white under surface, no feeling of pinprick on burned skin

Severe burns can cause large amounts of fluid loss, as well as infections. Burns to the face are particularly troublesome because associated damage to the lungs, which can occur if hot air is breathed in, can lead to breathing difficulties. Electrical burns may look less severe than they are because some of the damage is to internal organs.

Chest Pain

What it feels like: varies from a dull ache, to tenderness, to a sharp, searing pain anywhere in the chest.

What can make it worse: swallowing, coughing, deep breathing, movement, cold weather, sexual intercourse, anxiety, eating.

What can make it better: food, antacids, nitroglycerin, rest, massage of the painful area.

Your Doctor Visit

What your doctor will ask you about: heart palpitations, anxiety, depression, light-headedness, numbness or tingling in your hands or around your mouth, fever, chills, sweating, coughing, coughing up blood or mucus, feeling short of breath, tenderness, trouble swallowing, nausea, vomiting, swelling or pain in the legs, changes in weight, pregnancy, smoking. Your doctor will also want to know if you've ever had a stress test (usually an electrocardiogram [EKG] while exercising on a treadmill), or have been treated for heart trouble with medications or heart surgery.

Your doctor will want to know if you or anyone in your family has had any of these conditions: lung disease, asthma, chest surgery or injury, cardiovascular disease, high blood pressure, diabetes, elevated levels of cholesterol or fat in the blood, angina, phlebitis, emotional problems, obesity, congestive heart failure, heart attack, smoking.

Your doctor will want to know if you began feeling chest pain after chest injury or another specific event, or if the pain is frequently associated with eating, particular stressful events, or heavy exertion.

Your doctor will want to know if you're taking any of these medications: oral contraceptives, diuretics ("water pills"), digitalis, bronchodilators, nitroglycerin, tranquilizers, sedatives, antacids, or blood pressure medications such as beta-blockers, calcium channel agents, and antiarrhythmics.

Your doctor will do a physical examination including the following: temperature, weight, blood pressure, pulse, listening to your chest with a stethoscope, listening to your heart with a stethoscope, examining your legs for tenderness, warmth, or swelling, electrocardiogram.

Your doctor may do the following blood tests: blood count, testing for heart enzymes.

WHAT CAN CAUSE CHEST PAIN, AND WHAT IS TYPICAL FOR EACH CAUSE?		
CAUSE	**WHAT IS IT?**	**TYPICAL SYMPTOMS**
Chest wall ache	Pain in the chest wall	Tenderness in the chest wall, often worsening with movement or deep breathing, and possibly resulting from injury or a bout of violent coughing
Rib fracture	A crack in one of the ribs	Tenderness over the fracture, often accompanied by the sound or sensation of grating and crackling
Neck pain	Pain in the neck that radiates to the chest	Chest or arm pain that worsens when moving or putting pressure on the neck
Heartburn	Also known as GERD (GastroEsophageal Reflux Disease), the movement of stomach acid up into and through the esophagus, which connects the throat to the stomach; can lead to ulcer (see below)	Burning upper abdominal pain, worse when lying flat or bending over, particularly soon after meals, relieved by antacids or sitting upright

**WHAT CAN CAUSE CHEST PAIN,
AND WHAT IS TYPICAL FOR EACH CAUSE? (CONTINUED)**

CAUSE	WHAT IS IT?	TYPICAL SYMPTOMS
Ulcer	Severe irritation of the stomach or intestinal lining	Burning upper abdominal pain that is worse when lying down, sometimes relieved by antacids and made worse by aspirin or drugs such as ibuprofen
Cholecystitis	Gallstones	Fever, right upper abdominal pain, sometimes pain in right shoulder, nausea, vomiting, chills, sometimes jaundice (skin taking on a yellowish appearance), dark urine
Arthritis/bursitis	Inflammation in or around the joints	Tenderness in the shoulder, ribs, or muscles, often in the lower chest, may result after prolonged coughing
Angina pectoris	Sudden spasms of chest pain caused by lack of oxygen to the heart muscles	Chest pain behind the breastbone, aggravated by exertion and relieved by rest; pain may radiate to the left arm
Heart attack	Blockage in one of the arteries feeding the heart, leading to death of part of the heart muscle	Severe, often crushing pain behind the breastbone, sometimes with sweating, nausea, or vomiting
Crescendo angina (preinfarction angina)	A more severe form of angina pectoris (see above)	Attacks of angina (see above) that occur more frequently, or become more severe over time
Pneumonia	An infection of the lungs	Fever, chills, shaking, coughing up blood or mucus, sharp chest pain
Pneumothorax	"Collapsed lung": an accumulation of air between the lungs and chest wall	Sudden onset of breathing difficulties, sharp chest pain

**WHAT CAN CAUSE CHEST PAIN,
AND WHAT IS TYPICAL FOR EACH CAUSE? (CONTINUED)**

CAUSE	WHAT IS IT?	TYPICAL SYMPTOMS
Pulmonary embolus	A blood clot blocking the flow of blood to the lungs	Sudden onset of breathing difficulties, dull chest pain, sweating, light-headedness, apprehension, cough, coughing up blood, swelling or tenderness in the calves
Pleuritis	Inflammation of the outer layer of the lungs	Sharp pain anywhere in the chest, often aggravated by deep breathing, coughing, or movement
Pericarditis	Inflammation of the sac surrounding the heart	Pain over the heart or behind the breastbone, often aggravated by deep breathing, coughing, or movement
Dissecting thoracic aortic aneurysm	A tear of the aorta, the largest blood vessel in the body, which comes directly out of the heart	Searing chest pain that can start between the shoulder blades, abdominal pain
Lung tumor	Cancer of the lungs	Changes in coughing patterns, coughing up blood, chest ache, more common in smokers
Esophageal spasm	A contraction of the muscles in the esophagus	Severe pain behind the breastbone that is often relieved by eating, difficulty swallowing
Esophageal tear	A tearing of the muscles in the esophagus	Sudden and severe pain behind the lower breastbone, vomiting, sweating, often a result of a neck wound
Esophageal stricture	A constriction of the esophagus, which connects the throat to the stomach, that doesn't let food pass	Chronic pain behind the breastbone, food regurgitation, heartburn (see above)

WHAT CAN CAUSE CHEST PAIN, AND WHAT IS TYPICAL FOR EACH CAUSE? *(CONTINUED)*		
CAUSE	**WHAT IS IT?**	**TYPICAL SYMPTOMS**
Esophageal cancer	Abnormal cell growth in the esophagus	Feeling like food "sticks" in the throat or causes pain, weight loss, malnutrition

Confusion

What it feels like: feeling unclear as to what is going on around you, often accompanied by disorientation, difficulty maintaining attention, loss of memory, disordered or illogical thoughts.

What can make it worse: head injury, recent intake of alcohol or drugs, recent end to alcohol or drug habit, recent disease, changes in your environment, such as your job, home, or relationships.

Your Doctor Visit

What your doctor will ask you — or your caretaker — about: changes in attention span, changes in mood or the ability to concentrate, hallucinations, lethargy or stupor, excessive activity, changes in sensation or the ability to move extremities, headache, fever, vomiting, breathing trouble.

Your doctor will want to know if you or anyone in your family has had any of these conditions: chronic medical or nervous system disease, recent surgery or childbirth, alcoholism or drug abuse, history of emotional problems or psychiatric hospitalizations.

Your doctor will ask you about your ability to remember time, place, persons, and recent events, and will likely want to speak with a person who knows you well.

Your doctor will want to know if you're taking any of these medications: barbiturates, tranquilizers, antidepressants, amphetamines, steroids, atropine or belladonna, alcohol, marijuana, LSD, mescaline, cocaine, or other illicit drugs.

Your doctor will do a physical examination including the following: blood pressure, pulse, temperature, breathing rate, mental status exam including orientation and simple calculations, thorough eye exam, checking neck for stiffness and thyroid enlargement, listening to your chest and heart with a stethoscope, pushing on your abdomen, rectal exam, testing stool for blood, checking limbs for swelling and discoloration, thorough skin exam, thorough nervous system exam.

WHAT ARE THE DIFFERENT KINDS OF CONFUSION, AND WHAT IS TYPICAL FOR EACH TYPE?		
TYPE	WHAT IS IT?	TYPICAL SYMPTOMS
Delirium	Confused state resulting from underlying disease such as alcoholism, or the sudden worsening of diseases such as diabetes, or from medications	Disorientation, difficulty maintaining attention, going in and out of consciousness, hyperactivity, hallucinations; may include stupor (difficulty staying awake)
Dementia, including Alzheimer's disease, Pick's disease (similar to Alzheimer's), and senile dementia, but can also be caused by underlying brain problems	Gradual loss of memory and intellectual function	Memory loss, inability to perform simple calculations; changes in reflexes often occur in severe dementia
Psychosis	Loss of grip on reality; typical in schizophrenia and following use of drugs such as LSD	Disordered or illogical thoughts, typically no disorientation nor impaired intellect

Constipation (Adult)

What it feels like: an inability to have regular and easy bowel movements, often associated with bloating.

In adults, the most common and treatable causes of constipation are the use of certain medications (see below), reliance on laxatives, and a diet high in carbohydrates and low in fiber.

Your Doctor Visit

What your doctor will ask you about: abdominal pain, blood in stools, pain with defecation, diarrhea alternating with hard stool, weight loss, anxiety, depression. Your doctor will also want to know if you have ever had a barium enema or a colonoscopy, and what they showed.

Your doctor will want to know if you or anyone in your family has had any of these conditions: colitis, emotional problems, diverticular disease.

Your doctor will want to know what you normally eat, and how many bowel movements you have each week.

Your doctor will want to know if you're taking any of these medications: laxatives, enemas, sedatives such as Valium, opiates such as Percocet, antacids, anticholinergic medications such as Benadryl, calcium channel agents for high blood pressure.

Your doctor will do a physical examination including the following: pushing on your abdomen, rectal exam, testing your stool for blood.

WHAT CAN CAUSE CONSTIPATION IN ADULTS?	
CAUSE	**EXAMPLES AND/OR SYMPTOMS**
Medication use	Anticholinergics such as Benadryl, antidepressants, calcium channel agents used for high blood pressure such as Norvasc
Laxative habit	Overreliance on laxatives until you depend on them to have a bowel movement (can lead to decreased defecation reflex, below)
Poor diet	Constipation-causing diets are those with high amounts of carbohydrates and low amounts of fiber (found in whole grains and raw vegetables)
Inflammation of the anus	Pain on defecation, anus is tender
Irritable bowel syndrome	Chronic history of anxiety in which loose stools and lower abdominal pain alternate with constipation
Decreased defecation reflex	A result of chronic use of laxatives or habitual constipation
Partial bowel obstruction	Recent change in bowel habits, can also alternate with loose stools

Constipation (Child)

What it feels like: an inability to have regular and easy bowel movements.

The most common cause of "constipation" in children is concern from caregivers that they should have a bowel movement every day—even though it is normal for children to pass stool as infrequently as once or twice a week.

Anxiety from adults about toilet training can also be transmitted to children, which can lead to constipation. In this situation, most children develop normal bowel habits within two years.

Your Doctor Visit

What your doctor will ask you about the child: vomiting, excessive urination, crying during bowel movement, change in appetite, abdominal swelling, blood in stool, soiling of underclothes, behavioral problems.

Your doctor will want to know how many bowel movements the child has each week, how many the child is expected to have, and what kind of diet the child follows, including what kind of formula, if any, is used, how it is diluted, and how much the child eats.

Your doctor will want to know if the child is taking any medications.

Your doctor will do a physical examination of the child, including the following: weight, pushing on the abdomen, rectal exam, thorough skin exam.

WHAT CAN CAUSE CONSTIPATION IN CHILDREN, AND WHAT IS TYPICAL FOR EACH CAUSE?		
CAUSE	**WHAT IS IT?**	**TYPICAL SYMPTOMS**
Rectal fissures	Tears in the tissue lining the rectum	Pain on bowel movement, blood in stool
Abnormal feeding (infant)	Infant formula is overly concentrated, or the infant does not get enough fluids	Weight loss, dehydration
Bowel obstruction	A block in the passage of stool through the intestine	Abdominal swelling, decreased volume of stool, severe constipation, vomiting, weight loss
Encopresis	Inability to control stools (after age 4 years)	Behavioral problems, soiled underclothes

Convulsions (Seizures)

What it feels like: losing control of your movements, an alternating pattern of rigidity and relaxation, sometimes accompanied by a loss of consciousness.

Your Doctor Visit

What your doctor will ask you about: a "funny feeling" before or after the attack, changes in vision or hearing, changes in your ability to move, headache, fever or chills, stiff neck, tongue biting, loss of consciousness, loss of bladder or bowel control, palpitations, trouble breathing, nausea or vomiting.

Your doctor will want to know if you or anyone in your family has had any of these conditions: diabetes, hypertension, alcoholism, birth trauma, previous meningitis or encephalitis (brain infections), epilepsy, drug abuse, severe head trauma, chronic kidney disease, stroke.

Your doctor will want to know if you experienced a head injury prior to the convulsions, and if you may have eaten or drunk poison.

Your doctor will want to know if you're taking any of these medications: alcohol, anticonvulsants, insulin, diabetes medications, blood pressure medications, sedatives such as Valium, antidepressants.

Your doctor will do a physical examination including the following: blood pressure, pulse, temperature, thorough head exam to check for injury, thorough eye exam, checking your mouth for evidence of tongue biting, checking your neck for signs of stiffness, listening to your heart with a stethoscope, thorough skin exam, testing reflexes and movement.

WHAT CAN CAUSE CONVULSIONS, AND WHAT IS TYPICAL FOR EACH CAUSE?		
CAUSE	WHAT IS IT?	TYPICAL SYMPTOMS
Epilepsy	A brain disorder characterized by recurrent convulsions	Recurrent convulsions, sometimes family history of epilepsy
Phenylketonuria	An inherited disorder that leads to an inability to process a substance known as phenylalanine; now tested for at birth with a heel stick	Convulsions associated with developmental retardation, malformations from birth; convulsions normally begin before 4 years of age
Tuberous sclerosis	An inherited disorder that involves the skin and nervous system; characterized by facial rash, benign tumors of many organs, and mental retardation	Convulsions associated with developmental retardation, malformations from birth; convulsions normally begin before 4 years of age
Birth injuries	Varied, include cerebral palsy	Convulsions associated with developmental retardation, malformations from birth; convulsions normally begin before 4 years of age
Brain injury	Trauma to the brain	Severe head injury usually causing a fracture or penetration of the skull; convulsions can begin months after injury
Low blood levels of anticonvulsant medication	The result of a missed dose or of taking a new medication that interferes with the anticonvulsant	No symptoms other than convulsions
Stroke	A rupture or blockage in the blood vessels supplying the brain	Sudden onset of paralysis in one or more regions of the body, typically with a loss of consciousness, more common in older patients; can then lead to convulsions

WHAT CAN CAUSE CONVULSIONS, AND WHAT IS TYPICAL FOR EACH CAUSE? (CONTINUED)

CAUSE	WHAT IS IT?	TYPICAL SYMPTOMS
Hypertensive encephalopathy	Brain disease caused by high blood pressure	Convulsions in people with a history of high blood pressure, often associated with headache, blurred vision, stupor
Infection	Examples: meningitis, encephalitis, brain abscess	Convulsions associated with fever, chills, headache, stiff neck, sometimes stupor
Fever (child)	Elevation of body temperature, generally above 102 degrees F	Convulsions that appear in children between the ages of 6 months and 5 years associated with a sudden elevation of temperature
Overdose or withdrawal from alcohol or barbiturates	Taking too much of the drug, or stopping completely after a long-term habit	In the case of withdrawal from alcohol, for example, convulsions occur within two days after you stop drinking
Brain tumor	An abnormal growth of cells in the brain	Sudden onset of convulsions; may be associated with severe and persistent headache, nausea, and vomiting; more common in older patients

Cough

What it feels like: varies from simple cough to coughing up sputum or blood, sometimes accompanied by other symptoms, including sore throat, wheezing, or difficulty breathing.

What can make it worse: cold air, exercise, dust, the changing seasons.

Most sudden cases of cough are caused by a virus, and last for less than three weeks.

Your Doctor Visit

What your doctor will ask you about: runny nose, sore throat, facial pain, sputum production, coughing up blood, trouble breathing, trouble breathing except when upright, wheezing, chest pain, fever, chills, sweats, weight loss, leg pain, or ankle swelling. Your doctor will also want to know if you've ever had a positive test for tuberculosis, or if you've had a chest X-ray, and what it showed.

Your doctor will want to know if you or anyone in your family has had any of these conditions: lung infection, cardiovascular disease, lung disease, tuberculosis, asthma, AIDS, heartburn, heart valve disease, bronchitis or bronchiectasis, pulmonary embolism, lung tumor.

Your doctor will want to know if you smoke cigarettes or have been exposed to tuberculosis or industrial dusts such as asbestos.

Your doctor will want to know if you're taking any of these medications: angiotensin-converting enzyme (ACE) inhibitors (such as captopril), beta-blockers.

Your doctor will do a physical examination including the following: temperature, weight, breathing rate, checking sinuses for tenderness, checking the throat for redness, listening to the chest and heart with a stethoscope, checking limbs for swelling or tenderness.

WHAT CAN CAUSE COUGHING, AND WHAT IS TYPICAL FOR EACH CAUSE?		
CAUSE	**WHAT IS IT?**	**TYPICAL SYMPTOMS**
Upper respiratory infection	Common cold and other infections of the nose and upper respiratory airways	Runny nose, sore throat, facial pain, general malaise
Bacterial infections	Pneumonia or other infections of the airways and lungs	Begin over a few hours or days, usually accompanied by coughing up green or yellow fluid, fever or chills, sometimes coughing up blood, chest pain, fever
Bronchitis or bronchiectasis	Infection or inflammation in the air passages leading to the lungs (bronchitis), or destruction and opening of the airways caused by another disorder (bronchiectasis)	Chronic cough, trouble breathing, coughing up sputum, symptoms worsening in morning
Asthma	Recurrent attacks of wheezing, coughing, and shortness of breath brought on by certain triggers	Dry cough, sometimes trouble breathing and wheezing, often aggravated by exercise, cold air, a recent cold, taking beta-blockers
Croup (child)	Infection of the voice box	Barking cough, wheezing, fever, hoarseness, typically appears after a cold, more common in children between 6 months and 3 years old
Whooping cough (child)	Bacterial infection that produces coughing spasms that produce a "whoop" sound	Fever, wheezing, staccato cough, nausea, vomiting, most severe in infants

	WHAT CAN CAUSE COUGHING, AND WHAT IS TYPICAL FOR EACH CAUSE? (CONTINUED)	
CAUSE	**WHAT IS IT?**	**TYPICAL SYMPTOMS**
Medication use	Captopril or other angiotensin-converting enzyme (ACE) inhibitors (to treat high blood pressure), beta-blockers	Normal
Heartburn	Also known as GERD (GastroEsophageal Reflux Disease), the movement of stomach acid up into and through the esophagus, which connects the throat to the stomach; can lead to ulcer	Burning upper abdominal pain, worse when lying flat or bending over, particularly soon after meals, relieved by antacids or sitting upright
Cigarette smoking	Damage caused by long-term habit	Coughing up small amounts of sputum; over time can lead to lung disease
Chronic lung disease	Diseases of the lungs such as bronchitis or emphysema	Trouble breathing, cough and coughing up sputum worsen when first wake up from sleep, more common in smokers or people exposed to industrial dust
Psychogenic	Psychological or emotional problems	Barking, loud cough, occurring more often in daytime
Tuberculosis	Infection by tuberculosis, most common in people with compromised immunity, such as patients with AIDS or who have had organ transplants	Fever, night sweats, weight loss, chronic cough, coughing up blood

	WHAT CAN CAUSE COUGHING, AND WHAT IS TYPICAL FOR EACH CAUSE? (CONTINUED)	
CAUSE	WHAT IS IT?	TYPICAL SYMPTOMS
Congestive heart failure, mitral stenosis	A condition whereby the heart is unable to pump enough blood to meet the body's needs (heart failure), or disease resulting from problems with a heart valve (mitral stenosis)	Nighttime cough, trouble breathing except when upright, ankle swelling, family history of rheumatic fever or heart valve disease
Lung tumor	Abnormal growth of cells in the lungs	Change in cough pattern, chest ache, coughing up blood, more common in cigarette smokers
Pulmonary embolus	Blood clot that blocks the blood vessels feeding the lungs	Chest pain, apprehension, sweating, feeling faint, coughing up blood, rapid breathing, sometimes history of calf pain or leg immobilization such as on long trips

Cuts and Scrapes

Your Doctor or Emergency Room Visit

What your doctor will ask you about: when did the injury occur, did it occur at work, how did it occur, was there loss of consciousness (for injuries to the head), was the injury contaminated by feces or soil, whether there was an animal (and what kind of animal) or human bite, whether you have any numbness on or difficulty moving body parts near the injury, whether you have difficulty breathing (if it was a deep wound to the chest), or abdominal pain (if it was a deep wound to the abdomen).

Your doctor will want to know if you have any of these conditions: diabetes, bleeding disorders, heart disease, immune system disorders, organ transplant.

Your doctor will want to know if there is a history of domestic abuse in your home.

Your doctor will want to know if you are taking any medications such as steroids or blood thinners. He or she will also ask when you last remember having a tetanus shot.

Your doctor will do a physical examination including the following: temperature, blood pressure, pulse, examine the injury for: size, crushed skin and bone, dirt or other foreign matter, sensation and movement of body parts near the injury.

Your doctor will probably not order any blood tests unless the injury is very deep or severe or there are other associated problems. You may need to have a tetanus shot (booster) or other shots (such as rabies) if your doctor suspects an infection, or to take antibiotics.

Depression, Suicidal Thoughts, or Anxiety

What it feels like: feeling sad or nervous for no apparent reason, sometimes manifested as changes in appetite or weight, "panic attacks," trouble sleeping, forgetfulness, or thoughts of committing suicide.

Your Doctor Visit

What your doctor will ask you about: changes in appetite, fatigue, dizziness, changes in sleep or sexual activity pattern, thoughts of suicide (including how strong these thoughts are and how you might commit the act), change in bowel habits, changes in weight, changes in your menstrual cycle, forgetfulness, unusual thoughts such as obsessions or fears, crying frequently, palpitations, excessive sweating, tingling of lips or fingers, whether the feelings of nervousness or extreme fear tend to occur at certain times, during certain events, or in certain places.

Your doctor will want to know if you have had any of these conditions: mental illness, alcoholism, drug abuse, sexual or domestic abuse, any chronic disease, past suicide attempts, history of severe trauma.

Your doctor will want to know if there is a history of mental illness or suicide in your family.

Your doctor may also ask you about any recent changes in your life, such as in your job or finances, and whether you have just quit smoking or suffered any personal losses, like the death of a loved one.

Your doctor will want to know if you're taking any of these medications: birth control pills; methyldopa (Aldomet); steroids such as prednisone; reserpine (Serpalan); antidepressants such as Prozac, Zoloft, and Paxil; sedatives such as Valium; thyroid pills such as Synthroid; amphetamines such as Ritalin; beta-blocking agents such as propranolol, which are often used to control high blood pressure. Many of these drugs can cause depressive symptoms.

Your doctor will do a physical examination including: a mental status exam, in which you will be asked if you know where you are and other questions related to memory.

Diaper Problems

What it looks like: varies from diaper staining to skin inflammation in areas in contact with urine or feces.

Inflammation of the skin covered by diapers is called diaper rash, and is caused by contact with substances in urine or feces. The rash can be aggravated by waterproof coverings of diapers, wearing a soiled diaper for a long time, and the use of certain ointments or creams.

Your Doctor Visit

What your doctor will ask you about: if the baby cries when passing urine or feces, if there is any discharge from the baby's urethra, nausea, vomiting, diarrhea, fever.

Your doctor will want to know: how often the baby's diapers are changed, if the baby wears cloth or disposable diapers, how many baths the baby takes each week, what soaps, powders, or creams are used to clean the baby.

Your doctor will want to know if the baby is taking any medications, and if there has been any recent change in the baby's diet.

Your doctor will do a physical examination of the baby, including the following: thorough skin exam, testing stool for the presence of blood, rectal exam, checking for discharge from the rectum and urethra.

WHAT CAN CAUSE DIAPER STAINING, AND WHAT IS THE CAUSE OF DIFFERENT TYPES OF STAINS?	
COLOR	**CAUSE**
Red (urine)	Eating beets, blood in urine, certain medications
Green (urine)	Excess of bile, concentrated urine, certain medications
Black (stool)	Blood in stool, discharge of material after birth, excess of iron in diet
Green (stool)	Breast feeding, infectious diarrhea
Red (stool)	Blood
Extremely pale (stool)	Jaundice (skin taking on a yellowish appearance), antacid use, too much fat in stool

Diarrhea

What it feels like: frequently passing loose stools, lasting a few days or even years.

What can make it worse: anxiety (if diarrhea is chronic or recurrent).

Your Doctor Visit

What your doctor will ask you about: changes in weight, faintness when rising suddenly, nausea, vomiting, fever, chills, abdominal pain, blood or mucus or pus in stool, malaise, muscle aches, joint pain, colds, skin rashes, back pain, anxiety or depression, changes in bowel habits, tenderness around the rectum. Your doctor will ask how long the diarrhea has occurred, how often you experience diarrhea each day, whether you can eat or drink without vomiting, and whether you have eaten meat or dairy products within three days of the onset of symptoms. The doctor will also want to know if you have ever had a barium enema, an X-ray of your abdomen, or any kind of exam in which a doctor inserted a small camera into your rectum. He or she will want to know about any recent travel to a tropical or subtropical country.

Your doctor will want to know if you or anyone in your family has had any of these conditions: ankylosing spondylitis, emotional problems, diverticulosis, known ulcerative colitis or regional enteritis, perirectal abscess, past gastrointestinal surgery, pancreatitis, anemia, diabetes, recurrent respiratory infections, cystic fibrosis.

Your doctor will want to know if you have been eating a lot of cereals, prunes, or roughage, which can influence bowel movements.

If your diarrhea began fairly abruptly, your doctor may ask if you are at risk of having caught a "bug" – for instance, if you spend a lot of time in day care centers or nurseries, if you share toilets with others, or if anyone around you has the same problem.

Your doctor will want to know if you have recently traveled to certain regions or countries, which can increase your risk of getting a number of conditions that cause diarrhea, such as traveler's diarrhea, dysentery, or giardiasis.

If the patient is a child, your doctor will want to know about her diet, and if she has recently changed diets, how much milk she drinks.

Your doctor will want to know if you're taking any medications, **including:** adrenal steroids, sedatives, tranquilizers, quinidine, colchicine sulfasalazine (Azulfidine), antibiotics (ampicillin or tetracycline), antispasmodics, Imodium, laxatives, antacids.

Your doctor will do a physical examination including the following: temperature, pulse, blood pressure, weight, looking inside the throat, pushing on the abdomen, thorough skin exam, rectal exam, testing stool for the presence of blood, pus, eggs, or parasites.

WHAT CAN CAUSE DIARRHEA, AND WHAT IS TYPICAL FOR EACH CAUSE?

ACUTE DIARRHEA

CAUSE	WHAT IS IT?	TYPICAL SYMPTOMS
Viral	Infection with a virus	Vomiting, malaise, sometimes fever, cold, sometimes pus, blood, or mucus in stool, typically lasts 2 to 3 days
Bacterial	Infection with a bacterium, such as *Salmonella* or *E. coli*, usually food poisoning	Often begins within 72 hours after eating food or drinking water that made others sick, pus and mucus often present in stool, fever, typically lasts days
Bacterial toxins	Eating food contaminated with toxins produced by bacteria	Usually begins within six hours of eating food that made others sick, severe nausea and vomiting, typically lasts up to 36 hours

**WHAT CAN CAUSE DIARRHEA,
AND WHAT IS TYPICAL FOR EACH CAUSE? *(CONTINUED)***

ACUTE DIARRHEA

CAUSE	WHAT IS IT?	TYPICAL SYMPTOMS
Giardiasis	Intestinal illness caused by the organism *Giardia lamblia*, usually after wading or swimming in freshwater streams or drinking contaminated water	Bulky stools, abdominal discomfort, weight loss, typically lasts days to weeks
Schistosomal dysentery	Intestinal illness caused by a parasite that can be contracted in tropical or subtropical countries	Can progress to fever, chills, cough, hives, lasts up to three months
Amebic dysentery	Intestinal illness caused by a parasite that can be contracted in tropical or subtropical countries	History of recurrent diarrhea, profuse bloody diarrhea, abdominal tenderness
Traveler's diarrhea	Intestinal illness typically seen in travelers to Mexico and Latin America; also called "Montezuma's Revenge"	Stools may contain blood, typically lasts up to 2 days
Malaria	Blood infection caused by parasites and transmitted by mosquitoes, mostly present in tropical or subtropical countries	Cold clammy skin, profound weakness, fainting, jaundice (skin taking on a yellowish appearance), typically lasts days with cycling fevers
Cholera	Intestinal illness caused by *Vibrio cholerae*, a bacterium mostly present in tropical or subtropical countries	Low blood pressure, sunken eyeballs, bluish tint to skin, typically lasts up to 7 days

WHAT CAN CAUSE DIARRHEA, AND WHAT IS TYPICAL FOR EACH CAUSE? *(CONTINUED)*		

CHRONIC OR RECURRENT DIARRHEA

CAUSE	WHAT IS IT?	TYPICAL SYMPTOMS
Irritable bowel syndrome	Alternating diarrhea and constipation, sometimes occurring during periods of anxiety	Cramping, diarrhea, constipation, with minimal pain, no fever, typically lasts days and recurs
Crohn's disease (See chapter on Abdominal Pain (Adult).)	Chronic inflammation of the intestines	Bloody and/or frequent diarrhea, occurs more often at night, frequent abdominal pain
Ulcerative colitis	Inflammation of the rectum and colon	Low-grade fever (less than 101 degrees F), some pain in lower abdomen, blood may appear in stools, which are small and not well-formed, sometimes weight loss
Malabsorption	An inability to absorb nutrients from the digestive system, a result of bowel surgery or pancreatitis (inflammation of the pancreas)	Large and foul-smelling stools that are lightly colored and oily, weight loss, weakness, typically lasts years
Medication use	Resulting from certain medications, including antibiotics, laxatives, Maalox, colchicine, quinidine	Typically lasts between weeks and months
Partial obstruction	Blockage in the intestines, caused by tumor or the impaction of feces	Abdominal mass, rectal mass, constipation can also be a symptom
Diabetes	Problems in the regulation of sugar in the blood	Long history of diabetes, often nerve damage
Giardiasis	Intestinal illness caused by the organism *Giardia lamblia* (see description above)	Bulky stools, history of drinking contaminated water, abdominal discomfort, weight loss, typically lasts days to weeks

WHAT CAN CAUSE DIARRHEA, AND WHAT IS TYPICAL FOR EACH CAUSE? (CONTINUED)

CHRONIC OR RECURRENT DIARRHEA

CAUSE	WHAT IS IT?	TYPICAL SYMPTOMS
Cystic fibrosis (in children)	A genetic disease in which children become more prone to lung infections and digestive problems	History of frequent respiratory infections, family history of cystic fibrosis
Celiac disease	Inability to digest gluten, found in wheat flour	Weight loss, usually begins after child turns 6 months
Allergy to cow's milk	Bodily reaction to ingesting cow's milk	Vomiting, bloody diarrhea, severe weight loss
Disaccharidase deficiency	Lack of an enzyme that acts on sugars	Begins soon after birth, diarrhea is watery, explosive, or frothy

Many of the conditions that can cause acute diarrhea and are typically seen in people who have traveled to tropical or subtropical countries can also cause chronic or recurrent diarrhea.

Difficulty Swallowing

What it feels like: varies from trouble swallowing liquids, solids, or both, to regurgitation, to pain with eating or drinking.

What can make it worse: eating or drinking.

What can make it better: bringing swallowed food back up into the mouth (regurgitating), taking nitroglycerin.

Your Doctor Visit

What your doctor will ask you about: chest pain, neck pain, throat pain, regurgitation, neck swelling, wheezing, hoarseness, cough, heartburn, difficulty chewing foods, weight loss, anxiety, depression, drooling (child). Your doctor will also want to know if you have ever had a chest X-ray, an examination in which you swallowed barium, or an exam in which a doctor put a camera down your throat to look at your stomach's lining.

Your doctor will want to know exactly where the food sticks in your mouth, if you have ever swallowed chemicals, or if you have ever had a tube stuck down your nose to reach your stomach for feeding or an examination.

Your doctor will want to know if you or anyone in your family has had any of these conditions: Raynaud's phenomenon, ulcers, hiatus hernia, neurologic disease, recent or recurrent pneumonia.

Your doctor will want to know if you're taking any medications.

Your doctor will do a physical examination including the following: weight, checking the throat for signs of inflammation or swelling, checking your gag reflex, thorough neck exam.

WHAT CAN CAUSE DIFFICULTY SWALLOWING, AND WHAT IS TYPICAL FOR EACH CAUSE?		
CAUSE	**WHAT IS IT?**	**TYPICAL SYMPTOMS**
Muscle disease	Problems in the muscles of the mouth and throat	Throat discomfort, coughing due to swallowing air
Neurologic disease	A disease of the nervous system that affects mouth and throat functioning	Throat discomfort, coughing due to swallowing air
Inflammation	Inflammation in throat structures, including the tonsils; may involve infections such as strep or pharyngitis	Severe sore throat, swallowing may be painful, drooling (child)
Globus hystericus	Mental disorder in which you feel as if you are choking	No difficulty swallowing, sensation of a "lump in the throat"
Achalasia	Condition in which the tube that leads from the throat to the stomach is unable to relax	Regurgitation after eating or drinking, trouble swallowing, pain may disappear after regurgitation
Diffuse spasm	Spasms in the muscles of the tube leading from the throat to the stomach	Regurgitation after eating or drinking, chest pain with eating, pain relieved by nitroglycerin
Stricture	Narrowing of the tube leading from the throat to the stomach	More trouble swallowing food than liquids, nighttime regurgitation, recurrent lung infections, history of heartburn, maybe history of swallowing corrosive material
Scleroderma	Disease of the connective tissue	More trouble swallowing food than liquids, nighttime regurgitation, recurrent lung infections, heartburn, history of Raynaud's phenomenon (blood vessel spasms that affect the flow of blood through the body, predominantly affecting women and resulting in cold extremities)

WHAT CAN CAUSE DIFFICULTY SWALLOWING, AND WHAT IS TYPICAL FOR EACH CAUSE? (CONTINUED)		
CAUSE	**WHAT IS IT?**	**TYPICAL SYMPTOMS**
Diverticula	Small pouches that extend from the wall of the tube leading from the throat to the stomach	More trouble swallowing food than liquids, nighttime regurgitation, recurrent lung infections, foul breath, regurgitation of food many hours after meal, chest pain
Cancer	Unchecked, abnormal growth of cells into tumors in the mouth or throat	Throat discomfort, coughing due to swallowing air, chest pain, symptoms worsen over time, eventually regurgitation of saliva

Dizziness

What it feels like: a feeling as if your surroundings are spinning around, sometimes accompanied by nausea, vomiting, and ear problems.

What can make it worse: changing position, head-turning, coughing, urinating, standing suddenly after eating.

Dizziness is a common problem, especially in the elderly, in whom it is often associated with medication use and other conditions, and can increase the risk of falls.

Your Doctor Visit

What your doctor will ask you about: numbness in fingers and toes or around the mouth, anxiety or depression, headache, double vision, loss of hearing or ringing in the ears, numbness, loss of strength or sensation, lack of coordination, nausea or vomiting, palpitations, blood in stools.

Your doctor will want to know if you or anyone in your family has had any of these conditions: anxiety, depression, hypertension, diabetes, migraine headaches, cardiovascular disease, anemia, Meniere's disease, nervous system disease, ear disease.

Your doctor will want to know how long you have been experiencing episodes of dizziness, and how long each episode typically lasts.

Your doctor will want to know if you're taking any of these medications: aspirin, alcohol, blood pressure medications, diuretics ("water pills"), diphenylhydantoin (Dilantin).

Your doctor will do a physical examination including the following: blood pressure, hearing tests, thorough eye exam, thorough examination of your reflexes and movement.

Your doctor may also ask you to exhale while holding your nose and mouth shut, or to hyperventilate for 2 minutes and turn your head from side to side, to see if these activities cause dizziness.

WHAT CAN CAUSE DIZZINESS, AND WHAT IS TYPICAL FOR EACH CAUSE?		
CAUSE	**WHAT IS IT?**	**TYPICAL SYMPTOMS**
Central vertigo	Feeling as if your surroundings are spinning or moving	Weakness, lack of coordination, double vision, numbness, sometimes occurs after injury to important brain structures
Migraine-associated vertigo	Vertigo (see above) that accompanies a severe headache	Vertigo occurs before headache
Labyrinthitis	Inflammation in the inner ear	Sudden attack of vertigo (see above), nausea and vomiting, may recur, typically lasts a few days
Meniere's disease	Inner ear disorder	Trouble hearing, recurrent attacks of nausea, vomiting, ringing in the ears, vertigo (see above)
Positional vertigo	Vertigo (see above) that occurs after turning the head or changing position	Vertigo (see above) that occurs after turning the head, or changing position
Acoustic neuroma	Benign tumor in the nerve that connects the ear to the brain	Chronic and progressive loss of hearing in one ear, ringing in the ears, occasional vertigo (see above)
Hyperventilation	Rapid breathing	Light-headedness, no vertigo (see above), sometimes tingling in the fingers and mouth

	WHAT CAN CAUSE DIZZINESS, AND WHAT IS TYPICAL FOR EACH CAUSE? (CONTINUED)	
CAUSE	WHAT IS IT?	TYPICAL SYMPTOMS
Giddiness with sensory deficits	Dizziness or light-headedness accompanied by strange sensations	Light-headedness, no vertigo (see above), dizziness occurs when making a sharp turn or after eating, more common in the elderly and diabetics
Orthostatic dizziness	Dizziness that occurs when upright, caused by poor blood supply to the brain, a result of disease or medication	Light-headedness, no vertigo (see above), sometimes blood in stools, more common in people with anemia or heart disease or those taking blood pressure medications; may involve a loss of consciousness (See chapter on Loss of Consciousness.)
Dizziness during certain activities	Dizziness occurs when urinating or coughing, or after eating	Light-headedness, no vertigo (see above), occurs only with certain activities
Drug overdose	Dizziness that occurs after taking too much of a medication or drug, such as alcohol, aspirin, or sedatives	Dizziness, ringing in the ears
Eye problems	Double vision, decreased vision	Dizziness, double vision, or decreased vision
Chronic ear disease	May result from frequent ear infections	Decreased hearing, history of recurrent ear infections

Ear Problems

What it feels like: varies from decreased hearing to ear pain to hearing sounds that no one else does, such as ringing or buzzing (tinnitus).

Your Doctor Visit

What your doctor will ask you about: difficulty hearing in group conversation, headache, nausea, vomiting, fever, chills, ear pain, loss of ability to "pop" ears, hearing loss, ear discharge, ringing or buzzing in the ears, runny nose, sore throat, sensation of movement or rotation, loss of equilibrium, ear pulling (child), the date of your last ear exam, whether the pain is in one or both ears.

Your doctor will want to know if you or anyone in your family has had any of these conditions: hearing trouble, high blood pressure, nervous system disease, Meniere's disease, ear infections, severe head trauma, mumps.

Your doctor will want to know if your ear problems began after swimming or bathing, or after spending time in a noisy environment. Your doctor will also ask if there is a possibility you have an object in your ear.

Your doctor will want to know if you're taking any of these medications: aspirin, nonsteroidal anti-inflammatory medications, antibiotics, diuretics ("water pills"), quinine, lithium.

Your doctor will do a physical examination including the following: thorough ear exam, thorough tests of your reflexes and movement, hearing tests. During the hearing tests, your doctor may place a tuning fork in the middle of your forehead, behind your ear, or in front of your ear, and ask you about what you hear. Your doctor may also whisper behind your ear and ask what you hear.

If the patient is a young child, the doctor may do some exercises to see how the child responds to sound, his name, or simple words.

	WHAT CAN CAUSE HEARING PROBLEMS, AND WHAT IS TYPICAL FOR EACH CAUSE?	

HEARING LOSS OR DIFFICULTY

CAUSE	WHAT IS IT?	TYPICAL SYMPTOMS
Otosclerosis	Overgrowth of spongy bone inside the ear, gradually blocking the ear	More common in the elderly
Ear wax or foreign body	Overgrowth of cerumen, also known as ear wax, or presence of object in the ear	May begin suddenly or gradually, hearing returns when wax or foreign body is removed
Chronic otitis	Chronic inflammation in the ear	Foul discharge from the ear, loss of hearing (child)
Presbycusis	Degenerative changes in the ear	More common in the elderly, trouble hearing certain frequencies, such as in groups or on the telephone
Event-related hearing loss	Loss of hearing due to chronic noise, head injury, or the mumps	Trouble hearing certain frequencies, such as in groups or on the telephone
Acoustic neuroma	Benign tumor in the nerve that connects the ear to the brain	Trouble hearing certain frequencies, such as in groups or on the telephone, sometimes ringing in the ears
Ototoxic medication use	Hearing loss as a result of using medications that damage the structures used in hearing and balance	Tinnitus (see below), history of treatment with diuretics ("water pills") such as ethacrynic acid and furosemide, certain antibiotics or the anti-malaria drug quinine.
Congenital	Hearing loss present since birth	Sometimes family history of deafness, speech is often delayed

WHAT CAN CAUSE HEARING PROBLEMS, AND WHAT IS TYPICAL FOR EACH CAUSE? (CONTINUED)

HEARING LOSS OR DIFFICULTY

CAUSE	WHAT IS IT?	TYPICAL SYMPTOMS
Tinnitus	Ringing in the ears	Ringing sound, sometimes associated with hearing loss (see examples above), sometimes associated with excessive aspirin use

Note: if you have experienced a sudden loss of hearing, refer to the section below. If you are experiencing dizziness, see chapter on that subject.

EAR PAIN OR DISCHARGE

CAUSE	WHAT IS IT?	TYPICAL SYMPTOMS
Otitis media	Inflammation and infection of the middle ear	Ear pain, ear pulling, or irritability (child), loss of hearing, inability to "pop" ear, fever, sometimes occurs after a cold
Otitis externa	Inflammation of the external portion of the ear, also known as swimmer's ear	Ear pain, often discharge, sometimes decreased hearing, fever, may occur after swimming
Acute mastoiditis	Inflammation of a bone behind the ear	Usually occurs after otitis media
Chronic otitis externa or media	Constant inflammation of the ear	Persistent, foul-smelling discharge from ear, little pain, decreased hearing

Excessive Drinking (Water)

What it feels like: believing that you drink and urinate more than you should.

What can make it worse: drinking alcohol or coffee, taking diuretics ("water pills").

Although it seems obvious, it's important to remember that drinking more than usual will cause you to urinate more than usual. Adults produce an average of 1.5 liters — about 1.5 quarts — of urine per day, and typically do not need to wake up in the middle of the night to urinate unless they drank coffee, alcohol, or a lot of fluids before bed. If you are urinating more frequently than usual, but not producing more than the average amount, you may have a urinary tract infection or a condition that obstructs the flow of urine. See chapter on Urine Problems for more information.

Toddlers who are being toilet trained often have to urinate frequently and urgently.

Your Doctor Visit

What your doctor will ask you about: anxiety, depression, headaches, breathing difficulties when lying down, pain or difficulty urinating, fever, chills, dribbling or change in the force of urine stream, excessive urination at night, excessive eating, swelling in your extremities.

Your doctor will want to know if you or anyone in your family has had any of these conditions: diabetes, anxiety, depression, nervous system disease, brain surgery or skull fractures, kidney disease, urinary tract infections, prostate disease, cardiovascular disease, liver disease.

Your doctor will want to know how much you drink, how much you urinate each day, and how often you have to get up in the middle of the night to urinate.

Your doctor will want to know if you're taking any of these medications: diuretics ("water pills"), insulin, or other medications for diabetes.

Your doctor will do a physical examination including the following: weight, temperature, blood pressure, pulse, thorough eye exam, listening to your chest and heart with a stethoscope, digital rectal exam, checking your extremities for swelling.

WHAT CAN CAUSE EXCESSIVE DRINKING OR URINATION, AND WHAT IS TYPICAL FOR EACH CAUSE?		
CAUSE	**WHAT IS IT?**	**TYPICAL SYMPTOMS**
Nocturia	Waking in the middle of the night to urinate	Occurs after drinking coffee, alcohol, or a lot of other fluids before going to bed, otherwise healthy
Diabetes mellitus	An inability to properly process sugar	Weight loss, family history of diabetes, excessive eating, nighttime urination
Psychological	Excessive drinking or urination resulting from a mental disorder	More common in people who have anxiety or depression, most can sleep through the night without urinating
Diabetes insipidus	Disease involving the pituitary gland	Insatiable and constant thirst, urine output often exceeds 5 liters per day, may appear after head trauma, nervous system disease, or brain surgery
Diuretic therapy	Use of medications that increase urination	Nighttime urination, use of diuretics (common in people with heart disease or high blood pressure)
Chronic renal disease	Kidney problems	History of kidney problems, nighttime urination, weakness, feeling faint upon standing

	WHAT CAN CAUSE EXCESSIVE DRINKING OR URINATION, AND WHAT IS TYPICAL FOR EACH CAUSE? (CONTINUED)	
CAUSE	WHAT IS IT?	TYPICAL SYMPTOMS
Partial urethral obstruction	A blockage in the tube that drains urine from the bladder, usually the result of prostate problems	Nighttime urination, more common in older men, difficulty initiating urination, frequent urination, dribbling, decrease in the force of urine stream

Excessive drinking and urination can also occur as a result of heart failure or severe forms of liver or kidney disease. See your doctor if you have these conditions and are having trouble breathing when not upright, or experiencing ankle swelling.

Eye Problems

What it feels like: varies from eye pain to double, poor, or blurred vision.

What can make it worse: looking in a particular direction, wearing contact lenses, eye injury, the presence of an object in the eye.

Important: Never try to remove a foreign object that may be deeply imbedded in the eye. If you have exposed your eyes to chemicals, make sure to wash them out thoroughly before doing anything else. If you are experiencing sudden blindness or eye injury, seek medical attention as soon as possible.

Your Doctor Visit

What your doctor will ask you about: blurry or loss of vision, eye pain, eye redness or discharge, intolerance to light, double vision, tearing, dryness, irritation, or swelling in the eyelid, seeing halos around lights, headache, the date of your last eye exam, protuberance of eyes, trouble speaking, steadiness on feet, any other changes in movement or your senses.

If you are experiencing double vision, your doctor will want to know if the double vision is occurring in one or both eyes, if you see it everywhere you look, if it is constant, when it began, and whether its onset coincided with injury to the head or eye.

Your doctor will want to know if you or anyone in your family has had any of these conditions: thyroid disease, diabetes, high blood pressure, nervous system disease, heart disease, previous eye disease, migraine headaches, allergies, glaucoma, "cross-eyes," "wall-eyes."

Your doctor will want to know if you have been exposed to any dust, metal work, or toxins, such as wood alcohol or smog.

Your doctor will want to know if you're taking any of these medications: eye drops, eye ointment, adrenal steroids, the antipsychotic thioridazine (Mellaril), the malaria medication chloroquine, the antibiotic ethambutol (Myambutol). Your doctor will also want to know if you wear contact lenses.

Your doctor will do a physical examination including the following: blood pressure, tests of your reflexes and movement, thorough eye exam. As part of the eye exam, your doctor may ask you to look at a distant point and cover then uncover one eye, or to look at a chart through a pinhole. Your doctor may also check under your eyelids, or use an instrument to check pressure in your eyeball. Depending on your symptoms, he or she may order a CT scan or MRI of your head.

WHAT CAN CAUSE EYE PROBLEMS, AND WHAT IS TYPICAL FOR EACH CAUSE?

DOUBLE VISION

CAUSE	WHAT IS IT?	TYPICAL SYMPTOMS
Eye muscle impairments	Problems in the eye muscles, resulting from a tumor, trauma, or thyroid problems, can also occur after injury	Protruding eyeballs, eye pain, double vision appears when looking in certain directions
Strabismus	Lack of coordination between the two eyeballs	"Cross-eyes," "wall-eyes," squinting, may worsen when tired, poor vision in one eye, sometimes family history of problem
Intracranial aneurysm or stroke	Abnormal ballooning of the blood vessels in the brain	Headache, pain behind the eye
Diabetes	An inability to process sugar correctly	Headache, pain behind the eye
Brain stem disease	Problems affecting the structure that links the brain to the spinal cord	Trouble walking, trouble speaking, vertigo (see chapter on Dizziness), movement problems

**WHAT CAN CAUSE EYE PROBLEMS,
AND WHAT IS TYPICAL FOR EACH CAUSE? (CONTINUED)**

DOUBLE VISION

CAUSE	WHAT IS IT?	TYPICAL SYMPTOMS
Myasthenia gravis	Autoimmune disease that causes muscle weakness	Muscle weakness, trouble talking, double vision that worsens as the day progresses, sometimes drooping of the eyelid
Pituitary tumor	Unchecked growth of cells in the pituitary gland, which is right above the nerves that travel between the eyes and the brain	Double vision, sometimes lack of vision in certain spots, sometimes associated with unusual growth or other problems

EMERGENCIES

CAUSE	WHAT IS IT?	TYPICAL SYMPTOMS
Sudden blindness	Sudden loss of vision that can be due to blockages of blood vessels, damage to the retina, or, if temporary, multiple sclerosis	Vision disappears quickly and painlessly, sometimes feels as if a veil has descended over the eyes
Acute angle closure glaucoma	Sudden buildup of pressure in the eyeball	Eye is painful and red, headache, nausea, vomiting, blurred vision, halo around lights, may be precipitated by darkness or stress
Corneal ulcers	Infection in the layer that covers the pupil and iris, often occurs after scratch, use of contact lens, or presence of foreign body in eye	Eye is sore and red, blurred vision, intolerance to light
Chemical injury	Exposure of chemicals to eyes	Should be washed out instantly

**WHAT CAN CAUSE EYE PROBLEMS,
AND WHAT IS TYPICAL FOR EACH CAUSE? (CONTINUED)**

EMERGENCIES

CAUSE	WHAT IS IT?	TYPICAL SYMPTOMS
Penetrating injury	Object strikes eye	Sometimes pain, may occur after feeling only speck in the eye, hammering, grinding, or using power tools

BLURRED VISION, NO EYE INFLAMMATION

CAUSE	WHAT IS IT?	TYPICAL SYMPTOMS
Refractive error	The eye is unable to properly process light, causing blurred vision	Poor vision, nearsighted, vision improves when looking through a pinhole, vision may be worse in one eye, more common in patients less than 45 years old
Amblyopia	One "lazy" eye is unable to fix accurately on objects	Poor vision in one eye, eyes may turn in or out, more common in children
Cataracts	Clouding in the lens	Painless, gradual vision loss, more common in the elderly and people taking steroids or those with a history of eye disease
Presbyopia	Loss of elasticity in the lens	Difficulty reading, vision improves with distance, more common in people over 45 years old
Chronic blurred vision	Progressive form of glaucoma (see page 82)	Blurred vision, loss of peripheral vision
Toxic drugs	Caused by overdose of medications in eyedrops	Overly large or small pupils
Retinovascular	Problems with the eye blood vessels	Worsening of vision, more common in the elderly and people with diabetes, high blood pressure, or atherosclerosis

WHAT CAN CAUSE EYE PROBLEMS,
AND WHAT IS TYPICAL FOR EACH CAUSE? (CONTINUED)

INFLAMED (RED) EYE

CAUSE	WHAT IS IT?	TYPICAL SYMPTOMS
Simple conjunctivitis	Inflammation in the membrane that covers the whites of the eyes and lines the eyelids	Eyelid feels covered in sand, eyes burn and tear, blurred vision, mild if any intolerance to light
Acute iritis	Inflammation in the iris, the pigment surrounding the pupil	Severe intolerance to light, eye is sore and aches, blurred vision
Herpes simplex keratoconjunctivitis	Inflammation in the cornea or membrane that covers the whites of the eyes and lines the eyelids, caused by a virus	Intolerance to light, sometimes eye feels sore or covered in sand
Sexually transmitted diseases	Eye problems caused by diseases such as gonorrhea or chlamydia (see chapter on Sexually Transmitted Diseases)	Acute or chronic red eye, pus, only in people who are sexually active
Acute angle closure glaucoma (see page 82)	Sudden buildup of pressure in the eyeball	Eye is painful and red, headache, nausea, vomiting, blurred vision, halo around lights, may be precipitated by darkness or stress

FOREIGN BODY IN EYE, OR EYE INJURY

CAUSE	WHAT IS IT?	TYPICAL SYMPTOMS
Conjunctival foreign body	Object is in conjunctiva, the membrane that covers the whites of the eyes and lines the eyelids	Eye feels as though "something is in it"
Corneal abrasion or foreign body	Something has entered or rubbed against the covering of the iris and pupil	Pain, intolerance to light, occurs in people who wear contact lenses or had something fly into their eye
Blunt injury	Injury to the eye	Blurred or double vision

**WHAT CAN CAUSE EYE PROBLEMS,
AND WHAT IS TYPICAL FOR EACH CAUSE? (CONTINUED)**

LID PROBLEMS

CAUSE	WHAT IS IT?	TYPICAL SYMPTOMS
Sty	Painful, pimple-like object near the eyelid	Tearing, red and itchy lids, painful, pimple-like object on the lid
Allergies	(See chapter on Allergic Symptoms.)	
Blepharitis	Inflammation of the eyelids	Chronic red, dry, itchy, and irritated lids, crusty material in lashes
Chronic tearing	The eyes continually produce tears	Constant tears
Dacryocystitis	A blockage and infection of the tear sac between the inner eyelids and the nose, most common in infants	Swollen, tender skin near the inner eye

OTHER EYE SYMPTOMS

CAUSE	WHAT IS IT?	TYPICAL SYMPTOMS
Tic douloureux	Nerve problem causing facial pain and spasms in facial muscles	Jabs of pain, pain often occurs near the eye
Migraine headache	Severe headache	Seeing spots or flashing lights, occurs before headache
Proptosis	Eye sticks out, a result of tumor or certain other conditions	Eye bulges out, trouble seeing, double vision

Facial Pain

What it feels like: varies from headache and nasal congestion to pain located in parts of the face, such as the eye, tooth, or jaw.

What can make it worse: touching the area, chewing, lowering the head between the legs.

Your Doctor Visit

What your doctor will ask you about: headaches, recent facial injury, anxiety, depression, fever, earache, eye pain, visual change, nasal discharge, toothache.

Your doctor will want to know if you or anyone in your family has had any of these conditions: diabetes, headaches, migraine headaches, nervous system disease, recurrent ear infection, rheumatoid arthritis, glaucoma, sinus disease, dental infections.

Your doctor will want to know exactly where on your face you are feeling pain.

Your doctor will want to know if you're taking any of these medications: diphenylhydantoin (Dilantin), ergot derivatives (Cafergot), codeine, aspirin, other treatments for pain.

Your doctor will do a physical examination including the following: temperature, checking teeth for hygiene and pain, thorough head, eye, and ear exam.

WHAT CAN CAUSE FACIAL PAIN, AND WHAT IS TYPICAL FOR EACH CAUSE?		
CAUSE	**WHAT IS IT?**	**TYPICAL SYMPTOMS**
Acute sinusitis	Sudden inflammation of the sinuses	Sudden facial pain, headache, nasal congestion, runny nose, pain worsens when lowering the head between the legs
Acute angle closure glaucoma	Sudden buildup of pressure in the eyeball	Sudden facial pain, eye is painful and red, headache, nausea, vomiting, blurred vision, halo around lights, may be precipitated by darkness or stress
Dental abscess	Collection of pus in the gums, caused by an infection	Sudden tooth pain
Herpes zoster	Inflammation of the nerves in the spine and skull, causing redness on the skin; also known as shingles	Sudden facial pain, begins before, during, or after outbreak
Tic douloureux	Nerve problem causing facial pain and spasms in facial muscles	Jabs of pain, pain often occurs near the eye, may be brought on by cold, heat, or pressure over the "trigger" area
Temporomandibular joint pain — "TMJ"	Pain in the lower jaw	Pain on chewing, sometimes history of rheumatoid arthritis
Chronic or acute otitis media	Infection of the middle ear	Earache, decreased hearing
Migraine headache	Severe headache	Throbbing pain that can last several days, often experience typical "funny" feelings before pain kicks in, headache often centers in the front of the head, often preceded by nausea and vomiting, family history of migraine, may be caused by alcohol or stress (see chapter on Headache)

Fever

In adults, fever often accompanies illness, and may be the first sign you are ill.

In children, a spike in fever can occur in response to vaccination, or after a seemingly mild infection, such as an earache, cold, or flu. See below for other, less common causes of fever in children.

Your Doctor Visit

What your doctor will ask you about: shaking chills, changes in weight, night sweats, headache, stiff neck, ear pain or ear pulling, sore throat, chest pain, cough, sputum production, trouble breathing, abdominal pain, urinary frequency, pain or difficulty urinating, crying on urination (child), dark urine, bone or joint pain, skin rash or pustules.

Your doctor will want to know if you or anyone in your family has had any of these conditions: valvular heart disease, diabetes, tuberculosis, mononucleosis, AIDS, positive tuberculin test.

Your doctor will want to know if you recently traveled to another country, received a tick bite within the past two weeks, or had contact with someone with tuberculosis, pneumonia, strep, a cold, or the flu.

Your doctor will want to know if you're taking any medications, including steroids.

If the patient is a child, your doctor will want to know if he was wearing excessively warm clothing when his temperature was taken, and if he has been vaccinated within the past three days.

Your doctor will do a physical examination including the following: temperature, pulse, weight, blood pressure, complete physical examination, check head for sinus tenderness, thorough ear exam, looking in the throat, checking the neck for stiffness, listening to the chest and heart with a stethoscope, pushing on the abdomen, checking extremities for swelling or tenderness or redness, thorough skin exam, checking lymph nodes to see if they are enlarged.

WHAT CAN CAUSE FEVER, AND WHAT IS TYPICAL FOR EACH CAUSE?

IN ADULTS

CAUSE	WHAT IS IT?	TYPICAL SYMPTOMS
Upper respiratory illness	Cold	Sore throat, runny nose, cough, mild fever
Mononucleosis	Flu-like illness caused by the Epstein-Barr virus	Sore throat, fatigue
"Flu" syndrome	Conditions that produce flu symptoms but that are not necessarily the flu	Muscle aches and pains, nausea, vomiting, diarrhea, loss of appetite, malaise, mild fever
Urinary tract infection	Infection of the bladder or urethra	Frequent urination, pain or difficulty urinating, pain in the sides, sometimes blood in urine
Drug fever	Fever resulting from a reaction to a drug	Sometimes skin rash

SERIOUS, LESS COMMON ILLNESSES THAT CAN PRODUCE FEVER IN ADULTS

CAUSE	WHAT IS IT?	TYPICAL SYMPTOMS
Pneumonia	Inflammation of the lungs	Cough, coughing up green or yellow material, chest pain
Meningitis	Infection or inflammation of the covering of the brain	Headache, stiff neck

WHAT CAN CAUSE FEVER, AND WHAT IS TYPICAL FOR EACH CAUSE? (CONTINUED)

SERIOUS, LESS COMMON ILLNESSES THAT CAN PRODUCE FEVER IN ADULTS

CAUSE	WHAT IS IT?	TYPICAL SYMPTOMS
Intraabdominal abscess	Collection of pus within the abdomen, caused by an infection	Abdominal pain and tenderness, mass present in abdomen, recent abdominal surgery
Cancer	Unchecked, abnormal growth of cells	Fatigue, weight loss, masses
AIDS	Disease of the immune system, resulting from infection with HIV	Fatigue, weight loss, masses
Osteomyelitis	Inflammation of the bone	Bone pain, tenderness, swelling, muscle spasm
Septic arthritis	Joint inflammation caused by an infection	Joint swelling
Tuberculosis	Infection that primarily affects the lungs but can spread throughout the body	Cough, weight loss, night sweats, recent contact with an infected person
Connective tissue disease	Disease of the tissue that binds joints and other tissues together	Joint pain, headache, skin rash, chest pain
Bacterial endocarditis	Inflammation or infection of the heart, caused by bacteria	Trouble breathing, weakness, history of valvular heart disease, tiny red or purple spots
Thrombophlebitis	Inflammation of the veins	Leg pain, redness, swelling, tenderness
Rocky Mountain spotted fever	Disease transmitted by ticks	Recent tick bite, headache
Tropical infections	Any condition that occurs more commonly in tropical areas, such as malaria, leishmaniasis, Chagas' disease	Recent travel to tropical area; malaria's symptoms are cold, clammy skin, profound weakness, fainting, jaundice (skin taking on a yellowish appearance), typically lasting days with cycling fevers

What can cause fever, and what is typical for each cause? (continued)

In Children

Cause	What Is It?	Typical Symptoms
Wearing excessively warm clothing	An increase in body temperature as a result of wearing too much clothing	Fever subsides when clothes are removed
Bacteremia	Presence of bacteria in the blood	High fever with no obvious source of infection, more common in children younger than 2 years
Roseola	Disease marked by fever and the eruption of red spots	High fever that lasts three days, child is otherwise well, pink rash appears on the fourth day
Measles	Highly contagious disease caused by a virus	Cough, fever, pink eye, tiny white specks in the mouth, rash
Rheumatic fever, rheumatoid arthritis	Recurrent joint problems	Fever, joint pain
Skin infections, scarlet fever	Diseases that infect the skin, often producing rash	Skin rash, pustules, collections of pus on the skin

Foot or Ankle Pain

What it feels like: aching or burning pain in the foot or ankle.

What can make it worse: certain activities, such as walking, standing, or wearing shoes.

Your Doctor Visit

What your doctor will ask you about: joint pain, foot numbness, any previous X-rays or evaluations of the foot and ankle.

Your doctor will want to know if you or anyone in your family has had any of these conditions: gout, alcoholism, pernicious anemia, diabetes, rheumatoid arthritis.

Your doctor will want to know exactly where you feel pain, and if you experienced a recent injury to your foot or ankle.

Your doctor will want to know if you're taking any of these medications: gout medications such colchicines, allopurinol (Zyloprim) or probenecid (Benemid), the tuberculosis drug isoniazid.

Your doctor will do a physical examination including the following: a test of your nerves and movement, thorough foot and ankle exam, including checking for bone deformities, pain, swelling, range of motion, and pain on movement or weight bearing.

WHAT CAN CAUSE FOOT AND ANKLE PAIN, AND WHAT IS TYPICAL FOR EACH CAUSE?		
CAUSE	**WHAT IS IT?**	**TYPICAL SYMPTOMS**
Foot strain	Sore feet following certain activities	Foot pain, sometimes calluses, may occur after a change in occupation, shoes, or activity
Rheumatoid arthritis	Autoimmune disease that causes joint problems	Foot pain, pain in other joints
Ankle sprain	Injury to ankle	Ankle pain, tenderness, swelling in the ankle, history of twisting the ankle
Ankle fracture	A break in one of the ankle bones	Ankle pain, deformity, instability in the joints
Fasciitis	Inflammation in heel tissue	Heel pain, aching or pain after stress, tenderness in the ball of the heel
Achilles tendonitis or bursitis	Inflammation of the Achilles tendon or lubricating sac near a joint (bursitis)	Heel pain, tenderness and swelling in the Achilles tendon
Osteochondritis	Inflammation of the bone and cartilage	Pain in the heel and midfoot, more common in children between the ages of 4 and 14, may occur after injury
Neuroma	Abnormal, unchecked growth of cells from a nerve	Burning pain, pain worsens when squeezing the front foot
Degenerative arthritis	Joint inflammation	Chronic pain in the big toe, hurts with each step
Stiff toe	Stiffness in the big toe	Chronic pain in the big toe, hurts with each step
Bunion	Swelling in the big toe joint	Chronic pain in the big toe, hurts with each step

WHAT CAN CAUSE FOOT AND ANKLE PAIN, AND WHAT IS TYPICAL FOR EACH CAUSE? (CONTINUED)		
CAUSE	WHAT IS IT?	TYPICAL SYMPTOMS
Gout	Disease that causes joint pain	More common in men over 40 years old, acute and recurrent pain at the base of the big toe, sometimes pain in other joints
Neuropathy	Disease of the nerves	Sensation of burning or pins and needles, decreased feeling in the foot, more common in people with diabetes and alcoholism

Frostbite

What it feels like: numbness or pain after exposing part of your body to extreme cold.

What can make it worse: having had the exposed area wet while also cold.

What can make it better: removing the exposed area from the cold.

If your skin has been exposed to the extreme cold for a long period of time, and appears hard, pale, and insensitive to touch, you may have frostbite. While thawing, your skin may become red and painful.

Your Doctor Visit

What your doctor will ask you about: how many previous tetanus shots you have received, and if the exposed area is numb, blue, white, or painful.

Your doctor will do a physical examination including the following: thorough skin exam, to check the extent of frostbite and how well you can feel in the exposed area.

Skin that is white and insensitive to touch may be severely frostbitten. If you believe you have experienced severe frostbite, seek medical help immediately. If help is not readily available, place affected areas in warm—not hot—water, or cover them in warm cloths for 20 to 30 minutes. Wrap the affected areas in sterile dressing, try to keep them immobile, and drink lots of fluids. Allowing the areas to refreeze could be very dangerous, so only begin the thawing process if you are sure the area can be constantly kept warm.

Gait-Coordination Problems

What it feels like: varies from limping, tremor, or weakness to lack of coordination.

What can make it worse: darkness, trying to rise from a seated position.

People can feel unsteady on their feet if they experience dizziness when standing up. See chapter on Dizziness for more information.

Your Doctor Visit

What your doctor will ask you about: headache, tinnitus, weakness or changes in sensation, tremor, joint, back, neck, or leg pain.

Your doctor will want to know if you or anyone in your family has had any of these conditions: alcoholism, diabetes, any nervous system disease, chronic anemia, syphilis, cerebrovascular disease, cerebral palsy, arthritis or joint disease, hip disease, abnormal gait or coordination.

Your doctor will want to know if you're taking any of these medications: barbiturates, tranquilizers, anticonvulsants such as Dilantin.

Your doctor will do a physical examination including the following: blood pressure, checking muscle strength, watching you walk, testing your strength, sensation, and reflexes. If the patient is a child, your doctor may measure her range of motion in the hip and the length of her legs, and may ask her to stand on one foot or make a simple drawing.

What can cause gait and coordination problems, and what is typical for each cause?		
Cause	**What Is It?**	**Typical Symptoms**
Weakness	Weakness in the muscles controlling gait and coordination	Chronic problems, family history of muscle weakness, difficulty rising from a seated position, weak leg may waddle or exhibit a "flinging" movement, sometimes leg, neck, or back pain
Spasticity	Muscle spasms	May follow stroke or compression of the spinal cord, incontinence, mental retardation (child)
Minimal cerebral dysfunction	Slight brain damage	Normal intelligence, difficulty with challenging tasks, such as standing on one foot, threading a needle, drawing; only in children
Sensory ataxia	Lack of sensory coordination	"Stamping" gait, ankle jerks, usually worsens in the dark, sometimes history of syphilis or pernicious anemia, more common in people with diabetes
Cerebellar ataxia	Degeneration of a part of the brain that coordinates movement	Tremor, headache, ringing in the ears, unsteady or wide gait, may result from alcoholism, genetics, brain tumor, or stroke
Parkinson's disease	A degeneration of a part of the brain that coordinates movement	Resting tremor, difficulty starting movement, shuffling gait, poor balance, gradually worsens
Joint or limb pain	(See chapters on Joint Pain and Foot or Ankle Pain.)	

	WHAT CAN CAUSE GAIT AND COORDINATION PROBLEMS, AND WHAT IS TYPICAL FOR EACH CAUSE? (CONTINUED)	
CAUSE	WHAT IS IT?	TYPICAL SYMPTOMS
Congenitally dislocated hips	Hip problem present at birth	Limp, no complaints of limb pain, shortened leg, more common in female children between the ages of 1 and 3 with a family history of hip problems
Intoxicated gait	Results from alcohol intoxication	General lack of coordination, unsteadiness
Perthes' disease	Problems in the head of the thighbone	Hip or knee pain, limp, more common in children between the ages of 5 and 16
Slipped femoral epiphysis	Separation of the hip joint from the thigh bone	Hip or knee pain, limp, more common in children between the ages of 5 and 16
Hysterical gait	Psychologically induced walking problems	Feeling as if you fall frequently, staggering gait, injuries rare, associated with other emotional problems

Groin Pain

What it feels like: pain in the lower abdomen, sometimes a lump or swelling, which changes on movement.

Your Doctor Visit

What your doctor will ask you about: recent strenuous exercise, scrotal mass, change in bowel habits, abnormal pain or distention, need to strain to move bowels or urinate, recent onset of cough or change in chronic cough. The doctor may also ask about your sexual history, depending on the symptoms.

Your doctor will want to know if your pain is always present, or if it appears only in certain circumstances.

Your doctor will want to know if you're taking any medications.

Your doctor will do a physical examination including the following: thorough examination of the testes (in men) and groin, checking stool for the presence of blood, digital rectal exam, thorough tests of your nerves and movement. Depending on the symptoms, he or she may also test for infections.

If you are older than 50, your doctor may check to determine if you have conditions that can increase pressure within the abdomen, causing hernia. These can include prostate disease (in men) and gastrointestinal problems.

WHAT CAN CAUSE GROIN PAIN, AND WHAT ARE TYPICAL ASSOCIATED SYMPTOMS?		
CAUSE	**WHAT IS IT?**	**TYPICAL SYMPTOMS**
Groin muscle injury	Pull or tear of groin muscles	Pain and soreness in the lower abdomen and groin area, relieved by anti-inflammatory medications such as ibuprofen, and usually disappearing after a week to several weeks
Hernia	The presence of a loop of intestine outside the abdominal wall (but still inside the skin)	Bulge in the groin area that is bigger when standing and smaller when lying down, and can usually be pushed back into the abdomen with a finger.
Infection	Can include sexually transmitted diseases (See chapter on Sexually Transmitted Diseases.)	Swollen lymph nodes, other painful symptoms of sexually transmitted diseases

Hair Problems

What it feels like: too much or too little hair.

What can make it worse: recent childbirth, rubbing, pulling, or scratching at affected areas.

Your Doctor Visit

What your doctor will ask you about: itching, loss of pubic or armpit hair, menstrual irregularities, acne, voice changes.

Your doctor will want to know if you or anyone in your family has had any of these conditions: thyroid or adrenal disease, lupus, psoriasis or other chronic skin diseases, hair loss.

Your doctor will want to know if the problem began suddenly, or developed over time.

Your doctor will want to know if you're taking any of these medications: steroids, blood thinners, chemotherapy, minoxidil (a hair replacement treatment).

Your doctor will do a physical examination including the following: thorough skin exam, checking for rashes or other irregularities in the skin near the sites of hair loss or overgrowth.

WHAT CAN CAUSE HAIR PROBLEMS, AND WHAT IS TYPICAL FOR EACH CAUSE?		
CAUSE	WHAT IS IT?	TYPICAL SYMPTOMS
Male pattern baldness	Hair loss in men that occurs with age	Family history of baldness, widespread hair loss on scalp, begins in adulthood
Skin disease	Skin problems caused by infection, inflammation, or rash	Spots of scalp hair loss, history of skin problems or itching, skin lesions present in sites of hair loss
Fungus	Skin infection	Spots of scalp hair loss, bald spots with broken hairs, more common in children
Alopecia areata	Hair loss	Spots of scalp hair loss, areas are smooth and hairless
Hair pulling	Habit of touching or pulling at hair	Spots of scalp hair loss, history of pulling at sites of hair loss
Trauma	Widespread hair loss from scalp that follows a trauma, such as an infection, surgery, or childbirth	Sudden, often total hair loss
Medication use	Hair excess or widespread hair loss resulting from the use of certain drugs, such as blood thinners, chemotherapy, or minoxidil (a hair replacement treatment)	Hair excess or sudden, often total hair loss
Hormone deficiencies	A lack of certain hormones, resulting from suppressed activity in the pituitary gland or thyroid	Progressive hair loss, sometimes loss of pubic and arm hair, sometimes thickening of the hair shaft
Hormone abnormalities	Hormone imbalances, often caused by overactivity of the ovaries or adrenal glands, or from taking steroids	More common in women, hair excess, acne, menstrual irregularity, thickening of the muscles, voice deepens

Some people also develop excess hair for unknown reasons. Often, they are obese and have a family history of the same problem, but are otherwise healthy.

Hand, Wrist, or Arm Problems

What it feels like: varies from stiffness to swelling to pain in the hand, wrist, or arm.

What can make it worse: twisting the arm or exposure to cold (hand or wrist), lifting a cup, opening a door, or exertion (elbow or arm).

If you have injured your hand, try to keep it elevated to minimize swelling, and remove any jewelry if your hand is already swollen.

Your Doctor Visit

What your doctor will ask you about: weakness, numbness, swelling, pain, discoloration of the involved area, neck pain, pain in other joints, chest pain, nausea, vomiting, sweating.

Your doctor will want to know if you or anyone in your family has had any of these conditions: rheumatoid arthritis, psoriasis, past injury or fracture of the involved area, recent chest trauma or surgery, angina, or myocardial infarction.

Children can easily incur upper arm injuries if they are swung by their arms.

Your doctor will do a physical examination including the following: checking the affected area for swelling, tenderness, discoloration, dislocation or deformity; checking the strength of fingers, the grip, the wrist, and the upper arm; checking the pinprick sensation in all fingers; and a series of exercises to try to reproduce the pain you describe.

WHAT CAN CAUSE PAIN IN THE HAND, WRIST, OR ARM, AND WHAT IS TYPICAL FOR EACH CAUSE?		
CAUSE	WHAT IS IT?	TYPICAL SYMPTOMS
Osteoarthritis	Joint problems that develop with advancing age	Swelling, pain, and stiffness in multiple joints; in the hands, tends to affect the third joints
Rheumatoid arthritis	Autoimmune disease causing joint problems	Stiffness in multiple joints, swelling, pain; in the hands, tends to affect the first and second joints; can also affect the wrists and elbows
Psoriatic arthritis (See chapter on Skin Problems.)	Severe joint problems accompanied by rash	Rash, fingernail destruction, resembles rheumatoid arthritis (see above)
Bursitis	Inflammation of the lubricating sac near a joint	Elbow pain, swelling
Tenosynovitis	Inflammation in a thumb tendon	Pain at the base of a thumb, pain worsened by moving the wrist or thumb, pain reproduced by flexing the thumb or cupping the fingers
De Quervain's disease	Irritation or swelling in the tendons to the thumb	Pain at the base of a thumb, pain worsened by moving the wrist or thumb, pain reproduced by flexing the thumb or cupping the fingers
Dupuytren's contracture	Thickening and contracting of the palm tissue	Fingers frozen in a flexed position
Infection	Infection in the palm side of the hands, usually following a cut	Tender, red, swollen fingers or palm, sometimes pain when straightening fingers

WHAT CAN CAUSE PAIN IN THE HAND, WRIST, OR ARM, AND WHAT IS TYPICAL FOR EACH CAUSE? (CONTINUED)

CAUSE	WHAT IS IT?	TYPICAL SYMPTOMS
Epicondylitis	Inflammation of the upper arm near the elbow, caused by repetitive movements; also known as tennis elbow or golfer's elbow	Pain when opening doors or lifting, tenderness near elbow, pain worsened when bending or straightening wrist against resistance
Carpal tunnel syndrome	Compression of a nerve of the wrist, often a result of repetitive motion	Numbness, tingling, pain in the fingers, may worsen when bending the wrist
Pronator teres syndrome	Also known as pronator syndrome, this involves the compression of a nerve near the elbow	Numbness, tingling, weakness in the fingers, worsened by rotating the arm
Ulnar syndrome	Problems in the nerve that produce the characteristic feeling when you hit your "funny bone"	Numbness, tingling, weakness, worsened by pressure over the funny bone
Thoracic outlet syndrome	Occurs in people with an "extra rib" that squeezes the blood vessels and nerves near the collar bone	Numbness, tingling, eventual weakening of the grip, pain in the neck and shoulder
Raynaud's phenomenon	Condition in which the blood vessels undergo recurrent spasms	Fingers become painful, turn white then blue and red after exposure to cold, predominantly affects women
Shoulder-hand syndrome	Chronic pain syndrome affecting the shoulder and hand	Shoulder ache, burning pain in the hand, skin thickening, redness, joint stiffness, usually follows surgery or heart attack
Angina (See chapter on Chest Pain.)	Sudden spasms of chest pain caused by lack of oxygen to the heart muscles	Pain increasing with exertion, relieved by rest or taking nitroglycerin; shoulder and elbow pain can also occur, but are not the major symptoms

WHAT CAN CAUSE PAIN IN THE HAND, WRIST, OR ARM, AND WHAT IS TYPICAL FOR EACH CAUSE? (CONTINUED)		
CAUSE	**WHAT IS IT?**	**TYPICAL SYMPTOMS**
Myocardial infarction (See chapter on Chest Pain.)	Heart attack	Chest pain, nausea, vomiting, sweating; shoulder and elbow pain can also occur, but are not the major symptoms

Head Injury

Not all head injuries are serious. If you or someone you know has experienced any of the following symptoms of head injury, seek help immediately:

- Unconsciousness lasting longer than five minutes after the injury
- Trouble remembering events immediately before the injury occurred
- History of nervous system abnormalities
- Bone abnormalities in the skull
- Abnormal breathing after the injury

IMPORTANT: If you or someone you are with experiences a head injury and also has severe neck pain, do not move the head, because the injury may include neck fracture.

Your Doctor Visit

What your doctor will ask you about: stupor, neck pain, motor or sensory changes, discharge from ear or nose, vomiting, seizure, loss of urine or bowel control, tongue biting, pain in other parts of the body, cuts.

Your doctor will want to know if you or anyone in your family has had any of these conditions: alcoholism, cardiovascular disease, epilepsy.

Your doctor will want to know if you know what happened prior to your injury, if you were ever unconscious, and if so, for how long.

Your doctor will want to know if you're taking any of these medications: anticonvulsants, blood pressure medications, heart medications.

Your doctor may also want to speak with someone who knows you, to determine if you seem different from your usual self.

Your doctor will do a physical examination including the following: blood pressure, pulse, breathing rate, checking head and neck for discoloration or cuts, touching the head and neck to look for tenderness or bony abnormalities, thorough ear and eye exams, checking the nose for clear discharge, thorough examination of your reflexes and movement.

Your doctor will likely also ask you questions to check your mental status, such as whether you know where you are and what time it is.

WHAT CAN ACCOMPANY HEAD INJURY, AND WHERE CAN I FIND MORE INFORMATION?

Problem drinking	See chapter on Heavy Drinking (Alcohol).
Loss of consciousness	See chapter on Loss of Consciousness.
Convulsions	See chapter on Convulsions (Seizures).
Blackouts	See chapter on Blackouts.

Headache

What it feels like: throbbing, sharp pain or pressure in the head or neck, sometimes accompanied by nausea, neck aches, and muscle pain.

What can make it worse: head injury, anxiety, alcohol, certain foods, pressure over points in the face, placing the head between the legs.

The vast majority of headaches are due to muscle tension, fever, or infection. The brain itself cannot feel pain—the pain comes from stimulation of blood vessels, muscles, or nerves in the head and neck.

Your Doctor Visit

What your doctor will ask you about: history of unconsciousness, change in memory, motor or sensory change, nausea, vomiting, stiff neck, fever, ear pain, eye pain, change in vision, nasal discharge or stuffy nose, muscle aches or pains, anxiety, depression, seeing flashing lights or having "funny" feelings before the headache, results of previous skull X-rays, CT, or MRI.

Your doctor will want to know if you or anyone in your family has had any of these conditions: nervous system disease, previous skull fracture, migraine headaches, cluster headaches, emotional problems, sinus disease.

Your doctor will want to know if your headache wakes you up from sleep, if it occurs more often at night, if it began suddenly, or if it recurs.

Your doctor will want to know if you're taking any of these medications: aspirin, codeine, ergot, caffeine, steroids, oral contraceptives, sedatives, decongestants, any injections.

Your doctor will want to know where in your head you feel pain, and what the pain feels like.

Your doctor will do a physical examination including the following: blood pressure, temperature, thorough eye exam, thorough ear exam, checking sinuses for tenderness, looking for discharge from the nose, checking the throat, examining the neck for stiffness, thorough examination of your reflexes and movement, a series of exercises to reproduce the pain.

WHAT CAN CAUSE HEADACHES, AND WHAT IS TYPICAL FOR EACH CAUSE?

COMMON CAUSES OF HEADACHE

CAUSE	WHAT IS IT?	TYPICAL SYMPTOMS
Muscle tension	Tightness in the muscles of the shoulders, scalp, neck, and jaw	Constant band-like pressure that lasts days to weeks, pain often centers at the back of the head and worsens at the end of the day, triggered or worsened by anxiety
Classic migraine	Severe form of headache	Throbbing pain that can last several days, often experience typical "funny" feelings before pain kicks in, headache often centers in the front of the head, often preceded by nausea and vomiting, family history of migraine, may be caused by alcohol or stress
Common migraine	Severe form of headache	Resembles classic migraine (see above), often appears without typical "funny" feeling beforehand
Cluster headache	Recurring form of headache	Brief pain centered in the front of the head, occurs often at night, tearing, nasal stuffiness, sometimes go for months with no symptoms

WHAT CAN CAUSE HEADACHES, AND WHAT IS TYPICAL FOR EACH CAUSE? (CONTINUED)

COMMON CAUSES OF HEADACHE

CAUSE	WHAT IS IT?	TYPICAL SYMPTOMS
Sinus headache	Headache caused by sinus inflammation	Facial pain, nasal stuffiness and discharge, pain increases when head lowered between the legs, fever
Febrile headache	Headache associated with fever	Fever, muscle aches and pains, cough, sore throat
Cervical arthritis	Arthritis in the vertebrae of the neck	Pain in the neck and the back of the head, sometimes pain worsens with neck movement, more common in people older than 40
Tic douloureux	Nerve problem causing facial pain and spasms in facial muscles	Jabs of pain, pain often occurs near the eye, may be brought on by cold, heat, or pressure over the "trigger" area

RARE CAUSES OF HEADACHE

CAUSE	WHAT IS IT?	TYPICAL SYMPTOMS
Meningitis	Infection or inflammation of the covering of the brain	Fever, nausea, vomiting, stiff neck
Subarachnoid bleeding	Bleeding in the brain	Sudden headache, change in consciousness or neurologic function, vomiting, stiff neck
Temporal arteritis	Inflammation in the blood vessels of the brain	Pain in the base of the skull, chronic muscle aches and weakness, vision loss, more common in people older than 40 who have never before experienced headaches

WHAT CAN CAUSE HEADACHES, AND WHAT IS TYPICAL FOR EACH CAUSE? (CONTINUED)

RARE CAUSES OF HEADACHE

CAUSE	WHAT IS IT?	TYPICAL SYMPTOMS
Hypertensive crisis	Severe increase in blood pressure	Blurry vision, history of high blood pressure
Brain mass	The presence of a tumor or collection of pus, immune cells, or other material in the brain	Recent headache that does not resemble other conditions
Subdural hematoma	Blood clot in the brain	Headache and consciousness waxes and wanes over months, more common in the elderly, alcoholics, and people who have experienced head injury

Heart Pounding

What it feels like: chest pounding, feeling as if your heart were "flip-ping" or fluttering, also known as palpitations.

What can make it worse: exercise, intense emotion, standing.

Anxiety can produce symptoms of heart pounding in people with-out heart conditions. If you also lose consciousness, see the chapter on Loss of Consciousness for more information. If the heart pound-ing comes with chest pain, see the chapter on Chest Pain for more information.

Your Doctor Visit

What your doctor will ask you about: anxiety, depression, giddi-ness, weakness, tingling in hands or around mouth, fever, chills, chest pain, trouble breathing, loss of consciousness, pulse rate dur-ing palpitations, results of previous heart monitoring, the rhythm of heartbeats during palpitations.

Your doctor will want to know if you or anyone in your family has had any of these conditions: heart disease, diabetes, high blood pres-sure, thyroid disease, blood disease, emotional problems, alcoholism.

Your doctor will want to know how long each episode of heart palpitations lasts, if each episode begins and ends gradually or abruptly, and if you have experienced palpitations before.

Your doctor will ask if you smoke cigarettes or drink alcohol, and how much caffeine you drink.

Your doctor will want to know if you're taking any of these med-ications: antidepressants, digitalis or other heart pills, bronchodila-tors or decongestants, thyroid medications.

Your doctor will do a physical examination including the following: temperature, blood pressure, pulse, neck exam, listening to chest and heart with a stethoscope.

WHAT CAN CAUSE HEART PALPITATIONS, AND WHAT IS TYPICAL FOR EACH CAUSE?		
CAUSE	WHAT IS IT?	TYPICAL SYMPTOMS
Anxiety or depression (See chapter on Depression, Suicidal Thoughts, or Anxiety.)	Chronic feelings of a low mood or anxiety	Numbness in both hands, faintness, pins and needles around lips, trouble breathing, occurs in people concerned about their heart health, can be a "panic attack"
Drug use	Heart pounding that occurs after drinking coffee or tea or taking bronchodilators, antidepressants, digitalis, or thyroid medication	Occurs in people ingesting the listed substances
Cardiac dysfunction (See chapter on Chest Pain.)	Abnormal function of the heart as a result of heart disease	Occurs in people with a history of angina, heart attack, or congestive heart failure
Fever (See chapter on Fever.)	Elevated body temperature	Fever, chills
Anemia (See chapter on Weakness.)	Low blood count	Pallor, faintness, may occur after light exercise or standing suddenly
Thyroid disease	Abnormality in the thyroid gland	Inability to tolerate heat, weight loss, tremor

Heartburn

What it feels like: burning chest pain, sometimes gnawing.

What can make it worse: anxiety, alcohol, aspirin, certain foods or medications.

If you are experiencing chest pain other than heartburn, refer to the chapter on Chest Pain for more information.

If your pain is centered more in your abdomen, see the chapter on Abdominal Pain for more information.

Your Doctor Visit

What your doctor will ask you about: anxiety, depression, weight loss, weakness, abdominal pain, nausea, vomiting blood, tarry stools, results of any recent tests of the insides of your stomach, any successes with previous treatments or diets.

Your doctor will want to know if you or anyone in your family has had any of these conditions: abdominal surgery, liver disease, arthritis, chronic lung disease, alcoholism, ulcer disease.

Your doctor will want to know when and how you first noticed your heartburn, and how many times it has recurred.

Your doctor will want to know if you're taking any of these medications: aspirin, steroids (prednisone), warfarin (Coumadin), other nonsteroidal anti-inflammatory agents (ibuprofen, Motrin), indomethacin (Indocin), alcohol, antacids, acid-reducing agents (cimetidine, ranitidine, omeprazole), anticholinergics (such as Benadryl), sedatives, tranquilizers, antibiotics, coating agents (sucralfate).

Your doctor will do a physical examination including the following: blood pressure, pulse, pushing on the abdomen, checking stool for the presence of blood.

Some important factors to consider with ulcers caused by heartburn:

- Ulcers are caused by the movement of stomach acid up into and through the esophagus, which connects the throat to the stomach. Over time, this movement of acid can lead to ulcer, or irritation of the stomach or intestinal lining.

- Ulcers frequently recur. To keep this from happening, your doctor may ask you to:

  - Limit your intake of **caffeine, cigarettes, alcohol,** and certain medications.

  - Stick to your treatment plan once you experience any symptoms.

  - Report any signs that you may be experiencing gastrointestinal bleeding, such as overly dark stools, vomiting blood, or weakness when standing.

  - If, after avoiding the factors listed under "What can make it worse," you still have pain, your doctor may perform some additional diagnostic tests to understand your problem.

  - Some ulcers are **caused by bacteria**, so your doctor may give you **antibiotics** to cure your ulcers.

Heatstroke

What it feels like: collapse during extreme heat, sometimes leading to delirium or coma.

Someone with a mild form of heatstroke, known as heat prostration, will appear faint, have cold and clammy skin, and have a slight fever.

If a person with heatstroke falls into a coma, becomes delirious, or has hot and dry skin and a temperature of more than 103 degrees F, seek medical help immediately.

Your Doctor Visit

What your doctor will ask you about: headache, changes in thinking, loss of consciousness, nausea, vomiting, diarrhea, decreased urine output, sweating, cold skin, muscle cramps, bleeding.

Your doctor will want to know if you or anyone in your family has had any of these conditions: alcoholism, heart disease, high blood pressure, diabetes.

Your doctor will want to know how long you were in a hot environment, the temperature of the environment, your temperature at the time of collapse, and what you were doing when you collapsed.

Your doctor will want to know if you're taking any of these medications: alcohol, antihypertensive medication, diuretics, atropine medications, benztropine (Cogentin), phenothiazine antipsychotics such as Haldol.

Your doctor will do a physical examination including the following: temperature, breathing rate, blood pressure, pulse, thorough exam of your reflexes and movement, checking skin for sweating, color, and warmth.

WHAT CAN INCREASE THE RISK OF HEATSTROKE, AND WHAT IS TYPICAL FOR EACH RISK FACTOR?		
RISK FACTOR	**WHAT IS IT?**	**TYPICAL SYMPTOMS**
Dehydration	Not drinking enough water	Dry mouth, producing little or no urine, sunken eyes, more common in people taking blood pressure medication or drinking alcohol
Inadequate sweating	An inability to cool down by sweating	Lack of sweating when hot, more common in the elderly, diabetics, those with high cholesterol, people wearing too much clothing or engaging in excessive exercise, or people taking anticholinergic medications such as Benadryl and Cogentin, or phenothiazines such as the antipsychotic Haldol

Heavy Drinking (Alcohol)

What it is: your drinking patterns become a problem when you experience withdrawal if you stop drinking alcohol (see below), you develop an illness related to drinking, or it interferes with your social or work life; drinking to excess – a six-pack of beer in one sitting, or a fifth of a gallon of whiskey, for example, without becoming drunk – is also probably a sign of problem drinking.

For example, if you answer "yes" to any of the following questions, you may have a drinking problem:

1. Do you ever feel you need to cut back on how much alcohol you drink?

2. Have you been criticized for how much you drink, and has that annoyed you?

3. Do you ever feel guilty about how much you drink?

4. Have you ever had a drink when you wake up, to "steady your nerves" or cure a hangover?

Your Doctor Visit

What your doctor will ask you about: shakiness, confusion, trouble walking, seizures, vomiting blood, dark black bowel movements, abdominal swelling, jaundice (skin taking on a yellowish appearance), whether you've had a liver biopsy or other liver tests and what they showed, and whether you've ever had a test in which you swallowed barium for an X-ray, and if so, what it showed.

Your doctor will want to know if you have a family history of alcoholism.

Your doctor will also want to know if you or anyone in your family has had any of these conditions: seizures, delirium after cutting out alcohol, jaundice (see above), liver disease, gastrointestinal bleeding, depression.

Your doctor will want to know if you're taking any of these medications or drugs: anticonvulsants, aspirin, tranquilizers, antidepressants, marijuana, cocaine, heroin, other illegal drugs.

Your doctor will do a physical examination including the following: temperature, pulse, blood pressure, thorough skin examination, tests of memory, pushing on your abdomen, checking your limbs for tremors or shakiness, tests of brain function involving balance, eye movements, and reflexes.

WHAT HEALTH PROBLEMS CAN RESULT FROM HEAVY DRINKING, AND WHAT ARE THE SYMPTOMS?		
PROBLEM	**WHAT IS IT?**	**TYPICAL SYMPTOMS**
Tremulousness	Trembling or shaking	Irritability, flushed skin, stomach upset, sleepiness, occurs after several days of drinking
Delirium tremens	Delirium that occurs when you stop drinking	Fever, confusion, tremor, hallucinations, sweating, dilated pupils
Seizures	Convulsions	Occur within 2 days of when you stop drinking
Cerebellar degeneration	A type of brain disorder	Unsteadiness, abnormal eyeball movements, uncoordinated gait
Wernicke-Korsakoff psychosis	A brain disorder caused by a lack of thiamine (vitamin B1)	Confusion, memory loss, disorientation, abnormal eyeball movements
Neuropathy	Nerve damage in the extremities	Unsteadiness, numbness or burning in feet or hands

Hiccough

What it feels like: an involuntary and rapid intake of breath accompanied by tightness in the abdomen, often persistent.

What can make it worse: eating quickly.

Most cases of hiccoughs occur in people who are in otherwise perfect health, often the result of eating too quickly.

Your Doctor Visit

What your doctor will ask you about: abdominal pain, weakness, chest pain, new cough or change in cough pattern, trouble swallowing, anxiety.

Your doctor will want to know if you or anyone in your family has had any of these conditions: alcoholism, kidney disease, liver disease, nervous system disease.

Your doctor will want to know if you're taking any medications.

Your doctor will do a physical examination, including pushing on your abdomen.

WHAT CAN CAUSE HICCOUGHS, AND WHAT IS TYPICAL FOR EACH CAUSE?

CAUSE	WHAT IS IT?	TYPICAL SYMPTOMS
Rapid eating	Eating too quickly	Otherwise healthy
Gastroenteritis	Infection of the stomach	Nausea, vomiting, diarrhea, cramping, muscle aches, slight fever
Gastric distention (see chapter on Bloating)	An expansion of the stomach, either by food or gas	"Gas," discomfort
Lung tumor	Unchecked, abnormal growth of cells in the lungs	Change in cough patterns, coughing up blood, chest ache, more common in cigarette smokers
Advanced renal failure	Inability of the kidneys to function properly	Pallor, gradual lapse into coma, history of kidney disease
Encephalitis	Inflammation or infection of the brain	Fever, nausea, vomiting, stiff neck, headache, gradual lapse into coma

Hoarseness

What it feels like: a dry, scratchy voice.

The most common cause of hoarseness that has lasted less than 2 weeks is inflammation in the voice box, often accompanied by a cold and sore throat.

Your Doctor Visit

What your doctor will ask you about: cough, fever, sore throat, trouble breathing, wheezing, weight loss, coughing up blood, neck or chest pain, trouble swallowing, thickening of hair, cold intolerance.

Your doctor will want to know if you or anyone in your family has had any of these conditions: any chronic disease, alcoholism.

Your doctor will want to know if you smoke cigarettes, drink alcohol, or sing professionally.

Your doctor will want to know if you're taking any medications.

Your doctor will do a physical examination including the following: temperature, using an instrument to look into the back of the throat, checking the movement of the vocal cords, thorough neck exam, looking at the skin, checking your reflexes.

CAUSE	WHAT IS IT?	TYPICAL SYMPTOMS
Laryngitis	Inflammation in the voice box	Runny nose, sore throat, facial pain, general malaise; hoarseness lasts less than two weeks
Puberty	Period of becoming sexually mature, or capable of reproducing	Voice changes, occurs only in boys
Chronic inflammation of the larynx	Chronic inflammation of the vocal cords	Husky voice lasting years, more common in people who smoke cigarettes and drink alcohol
Epiglottitis	Inflammation of a structure in the throat that can block the air passages	Trouble breathing, drooling, sore throat, noisy breathing; occurs in children, particularly between the ages of 3 and 7 years.
Laryngeal nerve paralysis	Loss of function in the nerve that supplies the voice box	Progressive hoarseness, weight loss, cough, coughing up blood
Hypothyroidism	Decreased activity in the thyroid gland, which regulates metabolism	Progressive hoarseness, thickened skin, coarse hair, intolerance to cold
Tumor of the vocal cord	Unchecked, abnormal growth of cells in the vocal cord	Progressive hoarseness, more common in people who smoke cigarettes and drink alcohol

WHAT CAN CAUSE HOARSENESS, AND WHAT IS TYPICAL FOR EACH CAUSE?

Injury(Including Back Injury/Pain

What it feels like: an accident results in some type of bodily harm, or you have a pain that may have been caused by an unknown injury.

If the injury is primarily to your head, see below and the chapter on Head Injury for more information.

Your Doctor Visit

What your doctor will ask you about: the date of your last tetanus shot, the last time you ate before your injury occurred, details of the injury.

Your doctor will want to know if you or anyone in your family has had any chronic diseases or allergies.

Your doctor will want to know if you're taking any medications.

Your doctor will do a physical examination including the following: blood pressure, pulse, breathing rate, breathing pattern, examination of the injury and associated areas.

After your injury, your doctor will take certain steps to ensure that **you can breathe**, that your neck is protected, that you are not bleeding out of control, and that you are in no risk of **going into shock**.

If you have experienced severe head trauma, gunshot wounds, stab wounds, or blunt injuries to the chest or abdomen, your doctor will continue to monitor you closely for **months or even longer** to ensure you suffer no lingering effects of your injury.

See below for more detailed information on different types of injuries.

Head Injury

What your doctor will ask you about: unconsciousness, whether you remember what happened right before the injury occurred, vomiting after the injury, weakness, loss of sensation or coordination, whether you know who and where you are.

Your doctor will do a physical examination including the following: thorough head and neck exam, looking inside the ears, checking for clear discharge from the nose, testing reflexes, sensation, and strength.

WHAT ARE SOME FACTORS TO CONSIDER AFTER HEAD INJURY?		
FACTOR	WHAT IS IT?	TYPICAL SYMPTOMS
Neck fracture	A break in a vertebra of the neck	Neck pain, neck tenderness, occasional malalignment of the neck or paralysis in the arms or legs
Skull fracture	A break in one of the bones of the skull	Unconsciousness lasting more than 5 minutes, loss of memory for events that directly preceded the injury

Chest Injury

What your doctor will ask you about: breathing trouble, vomiting or coughing up blood after the injury.

Your doctor will do a physical examination including the following: blood pressure, thorough neck exam, checking for tenderness in the ribs, listening to the chest and heart with a stethoscope.

WHAT ARE SOME FACTORS TO CONSIDER AFTER CHEST INJURY?		
FACTOR	WHAT IS IT?	TYPICAL SYMPTOMS
Pneumothorax	An abnormal collection of air between the lungs and chest wall	Trouble breathing, chest pain

WHAT ARE SOME FACTORS TO CONSIDER AFTER CHEST INJURY? (CONTINUED)		
FACTOR	WHAT IS IT?	TYPICAL SYMPTOMS
Hemothorax	A collection of blood between the lungs and chest wall	Trouble breathing, chest pain
Cardiac tamponade	An abnormal collection of fluid or blood around the heart, compressing the organ	Trouble breathing
Flail chest	Severely labored and abnormal movements of the chest caused by penetrating injury	Trouble breathing, chest pain
Injury of lung tissue	Damage to the tissue of the lungs	Trouble breathing, coughing up blood
Airway obstruction	Blockage of the airways	Trouble breathing

Abdominal Injury

What your doctor will ask you about: abdominal pain, blood in urine.

Your doctor will do a physical examination including the following: blood pressure, pulse, pushing on the abdomen, checking for stability in the bones of the pelvis, digital rectal exam, checking stool for the presence of blood.

WHAT ARE SOME FACTORS TO CONSIDER AFTER ABDOMINAL INJURY?		
FACTOR	WHAT IS IT?	TYPICAL SYMPTOMS
Internal damage or bleeding	Damage to internal organs as a result of injury	Abdominal pain, tenderness, bruising, blood in urine, more common after a penetrating wound

Pelvic Pain or Injury

What your doctor will ask you about: blood in urine, inability to urinate, numbness or decreased strength in legs and feet.

Your doctor will do a physical examination including the following: blood pressure, pulse, thorough abdominal and pelvic exam, measuring leg length, testing reflexes and sensation.

WHAT ARE SOME FACTORS TO CONSIDER AFTER PELVIC PAIN OR INJURY?		
FACTOR	WHAT IS IT?	TYPICAL SYMPTOMS
Pelvic fracture	A break in one of the bones of the pelvis	Pain on weight bearing or direct pressure to pelvis, change in strength and sensation in legs, blood in urine
Urethral tear	A tear in the tissues of the urethra, which drains urine from the bladder	Blood in urine, inability to urinate

Injury to Arms or Legs

Your doctor may ask you to remove any jewelry or clothing that could become constrictive if your injured limb begins to swell.

Your doctor will do a physical examination including the following: pulse, temperature, sensation and movement in the injured limb, testing joints for mobility and stability, checking joints for swelling, testing for broken bones.

WHAT ARE SOME FACTORS TO CONSIDER AFTER INJURY TO ARMS OR LEGS?		
FACTOR	WHAT IS IT?	TYPICAL SYMPTOMS
Nerve or vessel injury	Damage to nerves or blood vessels in the injured limb	Loss of sensation or movement in the injured limb, pallor, coldness
Fracture or dislocation	A break in one of the bones of the injured limb	Loss of function in the injured limb, tenderness, swelling
Open fracture	Bone protrudes through the skin	Bone protrudes through the skin

Neck or Back Injury and Back Pain

What your doctor will ask you about: weakness, loss of sensation in arms or legs, pain in the neck or back, trouble moving the back or spine, blood in urine, inability to urinate.

Your doctor will do a physical examination before you are moved after your injury. The exam will include the following: checking neck and back for tenderness and alignment, looking for tenderness in the spine and along the sides of the body, pushing on the abdomen, testing reflexes and sensation.

WHAT ARE SOME CAUSES OF NECK OR BACK INJURY OR BACK PAIN?		
CAUSE	WHAT IS IT?	TYPICAL SYMPTOMS
Muscle strain	Reversible injury to the muscles that can occur after lifting heavy objects; this is the cause of about 70% of back pain	Sudden onset after strenuous activity, pain does not move to legs
Arthritis	Inflammation of the joints	Pain is usually present in extremities as well as back
Herniated disk	Abnormal bulging of the spongy disks that keep the spinal bones properly spaced	Difficulty moving legs, worsened by coughing or sneezing, may involve difficulty urinating, sometimes follows spine fracture (see below)
Spine fracture	A break in one of the vertebrae, often due to osteoporosis, which primarily affects women after menopause	Neck or back pain
Spinal stenosis	Narrowing of the space in the bones in which the spinal cord sits	Low back pain moving to the thighs (pain may be relieved by bending forward), thigh weakness, unsteady gait
Major neurological deficit	Injury to one of the nerves that comes out of the spine and travels to the extremities	Loss of sensation in the extremities, difficulty urinating

WHAT ARE SOME CAUSES OF NECK OR BACK INJURY OR BACK PAIN? (CONTINUED)		
CAUSE	WHAT IS IT?	TYPICAL SYMPTOMS
Spinal cord injury or compression	Damage to or constriction of the spinal cord	Paralysis, numbness, inability to urinate
Herpes zoster	A re-activation of chicken pox, also known as shingles	Pain is usually on skin in a narrow band around the body
Malignant tumor in vertebrae	A cancerous growth that has traveled from another part of the body into the bones of the spine	History of cancer, pain when certain bones of the spine are touched, usually severe and worsening pain
Urinary tract trauma	Damage to any of the organs that help funnel urine out of the body	Pain in the back or sides, blood in urine
Abdominal aortic aneurysm	Abnormal bulging of the largest blood vessel in the body – life-threatening	Extreme pain, pulsing mass in the abdomen, may be associated with weakness

Irritability (Child)

What it looks like: refusing to eat or perform expected tasks, fussiness, or other changes in behavior.

Childhood irritability can occur when a child feels badly because of disease or experiences problems coping with life changes or other aspects of his environment.

Your Doctor Visit

What your doctor will ask you about: headache, stiff neck, fever, ear pulling, salivation, nausea, vomiting, changes in appetite, diarrhea, crying when urinating, coughing, wheezing, difficulty breathing, skin rash, changes in weight, excessive crying, difficulty reading, attitudes toward school, hyperactivity.

Your doctor will want to know if the child has had any conditions or diseases, including: birth trauma, retardation, seizures (convulsions).

Your doctor will want to know what the child refuses to do, the nature of his irritable behavior, his medications, and how he acts differently from other siblings when they were his age.

Your doctor will do a physical examination including the following: temperature, height, weight, feeling the skull, hearing, eyesight, looking inside the mouth and throat, listening to the chest and heart with a stethoscope, pushing on the abdomen, testing reflexes and movement, testing developmental skills.

WHAT CAN CAUSE IRRITABILITY IN CHILDREN, AND WHAT ARE SOME ASSOCIATED SYMPTOMS?	
CAUSE	**ASSOCIATED SYMPTOMS**
Attention deficit/ hyperactivity disorder	Difficulty sitting still or paying attention, poor school performance
Autism	Bizarre or unpredictable behavior, failure to communicate
Obsessive-compulsive disorder	Frequent checking or repetitive behaviors
Meningitis	Fever, headache, stiff neck, squinting
Ear infection	Fever, ear pain
Teething	Tooth pain, crying spells
Seizures	Convulsions, uncontrolled shaking, loss of consciousness
Dyslexia and learning disorders	Difficulty reading and comprehending
Deafness	Difficulty hearing, or complete deafness
Skin conditions	Deforming skin conditions, shyness
Mental retardation	Extreme difficulty comprehending, low IQ

Joint Pain

What it feels like: pain involving one or more joints, which may extend to muscles.

What can make it worse: exercise, movement of the joint, injury.

What can make it better: rest.

For more information about pain in the hand, wrist, or arms, see the chapter on Hand, Wrist, or Arm Problems. If your pain is only in your foot or ankle, see the chapter on Foot or Ankle Pain.

Your Doctor Visit (shoulder or left arm pain)

What your doctor will ask you about: chest pain, muscle pain, pain in other joints, pain spreading to other joints.

Your doctor will want to know if you or anyone in your family has had any of these conditions: diabetes, high blood pressure, heart disease, past shoulder dislocations, or episodes of bursitis.

Your Doctor Visit (hip pain)

What your doctor will ask you about: ability to walk, low back pain, muscle pain, pain in other joints, pain spreading to other joints.

Your doctor will want to know if you or anyone in your family has had any of these conditions: sickle-cell disease, past surgery on or near hip.

Your Doctor Visit (knee pain)

What your doctor will ask you about: muscle pain, pain in other joints, pain spreading to other joints, pain on squatting or running up and down stairs, feeling of snapping, catching, or buckling.

Your doctor will want to know if you or anyone in your family has had any of these conditions: hemophilia, past knee injury or surgery.

Your Doctor Visit (calf or leg pain)

What your doctor will ask you about: muscle pain, pain in other joints, pain spreading to other joints, calf swelling or tenderness, low back pain, pain worsened by coughing.

Your doctor will want to know if you or anyone in your family has had any of these conditions: heart disease, chronic lung disease, recent surgery or prolonged immobilization, thrombophlebitis.

Your Doctor Visit (general joint pain)

What your doctor will ask you about: muscle pain, pain in other joints, pain spreading to other joints, fever, stiffness of joints in the morning, skin lesions, back pain, cough, runny nose, diarrhea, headache, finger pain, discoloration in the cold.

Your doctor will want to know if you or anyone in your family has had any of these conditions: rheumatoid arthritis, gout, gonorrhea, past trauma or surgery to painful area, rheumatic fever, genital discharge.

Your doctor will want to know if you're taking any medications.

Your doctor will want to know if your pain gets worse at the end of the day or if you feel especially stiff in the morning and, if so, for how long.

Your doctor will want to know how long your pain has occurred, and if you were recently exposed to deer ticks or strep throat.

Your doctor will do a physical examination including the following:

- **Pain in arms or legs:** checking for swelling, tenderness, deformity, discoloration or warmth, range of motion.

- **Knee pain**: checking range of motion in the hips, knee tenderness, knee joint stability, a series of tests to check knee function.

- **Shoulder pain**: checking tenderness, a series of tests to try to pinpoint the source of pain.

- **Calf pain**: checking tenderness, calf size differences, skin, pulse.

- **Leg pain**: checking range of motion in hips, pulse, a series of exercises to try to pinpoint the cause of pain.

WHAT CAN CAUSE JOINT PAIN,
AND WHAT IS TYPICAL FOR EACH CAUSE?

GENERAL JOINT PAIN

CAUSE	WHAT IS IT?	TYPICAL SYMPTOMS
Osteoarthritis	Joint inflammation associated with aging	Persistent pain in one or more joints, seldom in wrists or elbows or shoulders, occurs more commonly in people over 40
Virus	Joint pain associated with a viral infection, such as the common cold	Joint pain associated with flu-like symptoms, pain often disappears within a few minutes
Post-infectious arthritis	Joint pain occurring after some type of bacterial infection	Pain in at least one joint, history of infection with the bacteria that cause gonorrhea, history of discharge from the vagina or urethra (the tube that carries urine out of the body), fever, skin rashes, warmth and tenderness in joints
Gout	Joint pain caused by abnormal breakdown of substances by the body	Warm and red joints, tender and swollen joints, pain in at least one joint, family history of gout, tends to occur in big toe

**WHAT CAN CAUSE JOINT PAIN,
AND WHAT IS TYPICAL FOR EACH CAUSE? (CONTINUED)**

GENERAL JOINT PAIN

CAUSE	WHAT IS IT?	TYPICAL SYMPTOMS
Rheumatoid arthritis	Disease in which the body attacks itself, causing joint problems	Morning joint stiffness, pain lasts more than six weeks, pain on motion
Lyme disease	Inflammatory disease transmitted by tick bites	Warm and swollen "bulls-eye" rash, spreading rash, occurs only in people living in or traveling to areas in which ticks are endemic
Connective tissue disease	Disease of a major type of body tissue	Finger pain, discoloration in the cold, persistent skin rashes

BONE PAIN

CAUSE	WHAT IS IT?	TYPICAL SYMPTOMS
Fracture or dislocation	A break in or displacement of the bone	Occurs after injury, tenderness, swelling, inability to move affected limb
Steomyelitis	Bone infection	Fever, limp, bone tenderness, warmth in overlying skin

KNEE PAIN (ADULT)

CAUSE	WHAT IS IT?	TYPICAL SYMPTOMS
Meniscus or ligament tears	Tears to the tissues that help cushion bones and connect them to muscles	Knee buckling, locking of the knee at a 30-degree angle
Referred pain from hip	Hip pain that is felt in the knee	Hip pain, hip movement problems
Iliotibial band	Thickening of the tissue around the knee	Burning or tightening in the knee after running

**WHAT CAN CAUSE JOINT PAIN,
AND WHAT IS TYPICAL FOR EACH CAUSE? (CONTINUED)**

KNEE PAIN (CHILD)

Cause	What Is It?	Typical Symptoms
Hemophilia	Hereditary disease in which the blood cannot form clots	Heavy bleeding after minor injury, family history of bleeding, swollen joints
Osgood-Schlatter disease	Painful swelling in a region of the lower leg bone	Pain on squatting
Chondroma-lacia patellae	Softening of the cartilage in front of kneecap	Pain when ascending or descending stairs

HIP PAIN

Cause	What Is It?	Typical Symptoms
Osteoarthritis	Joint problems that develop with advancing age	Limping, occurs after age 50
Perthes' disease	Deterioration of bone in the hip	Occurs only in children, knee pain, limping
Necrosis of hip	Death of portions of the hip bone	Occurs at any age, more common in people taking adrenal steroids or those with sickle-cell disease

SHOULDER PAIN

Cause	What Is It?	Typical Symptoms
Bursitis	Inflammation of the lubricating sac near a shoulder joint	Pain when moving shoulder particularly when combing hair or lifting objects
Referred pain from neck	Neck pain that radiates to the shoulder	Ache in upper arm or shoulder, certain neck positions can worsen pain
Angina	Sudden spasms of chest pain caused by lack of oxygen to the heart muscles	Chest and arm pain, pain caused by exertion and relieved by rest or nitroglycerin

**WHAT CAN CAUSE JOINT PAIN,
AND WHAT IS TYPICAL FOR EACH CAUSE? (CONTINUED)**

CALF OR LEG PAIN, NUMBNESS, OR TINGLING

CAUSE	WHAT IS IT?	TYPICAL SYMPTOMS
Sciatica	Back pain that travels along a nerve into the buttocks, legs, and hips	Low back pain, leg pain or numbness, pain worsens with coughing
Chronic claudication	Calf pain caused by an inadequate blood supply	Cramps, fatigue with exercise, pain relieved by rest; heart disease is often associated with this
Acute embolus	Blockage in the blood vessels feeding the legs	Sudden pain eventually leading to tingling sensations on skin or paralysis, more common in people with a history of heart disease

BLOOD VESSEL DISEASES

CAUSE	WHAT IS IT?	TYPICAL SYMPTOMS
Venous thrombosis	Blockage of a blood vessel by a clot	Aching, tenderness, leg swelling, occasional chest pain or trouble breathing or coughing up blood
Venous insufficiency	Lack of blood flow from a limb that causes blood to pool	Chronic aching or heaviness in legs, elevating the leg relieves pain, brown discoloration of skin

Loss of Consciousness

What it feels like: partial or complete loss of consciousness, from which people either can or cannot be aroused.

Loss of consciousness most often results from head injury, drug overdose, or drinking too much alcohol.

Your Doctor Visit

What the doctor will ask about: fever, shaking chills, headache, sweating, tremulousness, convulsion, trouble breathing, cough, nausea, vomiting, painful or difficult urination, dark urine, recent change in urine quantity, change in sensation or movements.

The doctor will want to know if the patient or anyone in his family has had any of these conditions: any chronic disease, convulsions or seizures, emotional problems, nervous system disease, diabetes, high blood pressure, renal or liver disease, alcoholism, lung disease, heart disease.

The doctor will want to know what happened immediately before the patient lost consciousness, and how quickly he lost consciousness.

The doctor will want to know if the patient is taking any medications, including: sedatives, tranquilizers, insulin, opiates.

The doctor will do a physical examination including the following: blood pressure, breathing rate, pulse, temperature, thorough eye exam, checking the neck for stiffness, listening to the chest with a stethoscope, skin exam, checking extremities for swelling, thorough check of the reflexes and movement.

WHAT CAN CAUSE LOSS OF CONSCIOUSNESS, AND WHAT IS TYPICAL FOR EACH CAUSE?

CAUSE	WHAT IS IT?	TYPICAL SYMPTOMS
Blackouts (See chapter on Blackouts.)	Temporarily losing consciousness or vision, or feeling faint or giddy	Blacking out after standing, exercise, stress, or a particular activity like coughing or urinating
Seizures (See chapter on Convulsions [Seizures].)	Convulsions	Losing control of your movements, an alternating pattern of rigidity and relaxation, sometimes accompanied by a loss of consciousness, sometimes accompanied by loss of bowel or bladder control
Head injury (See chapter on Head Injury.)	Minor or severe injury to the head	Sometimes accompanied by loss of consciousness, neck pain, motor or sensory changes, discharge from ear or nose, vomiting, seizure, loss of urine or bowel control
Insulin overdose	Taking too much insulin, given to diabetics	May be preceded by tremulousness, sweating, headache
Drug overdose or poison ingestion (See chapter on Overdose or Poisoning.)	Taking too much of a drug, ingesting poison, or drinking too much alcohol	May be associated with a suicide attempt, abnormal breathing, fever, low temperature, changes in skin color, tremors, convulsions, or spasms
Meningitis	Infection or inflammation of the covering of the brain	Fever, nausea, vomiting, stiff neck, headache, gradual lapse into coma
Encephalitis	Infection or inflammation of the brain (e.g., West Nile virus)	Fever, nausea, vomiting, stiff neck, headache, gradual lapse into coma

WHAT CAN CAUSE LOSS OF CONSCIOUSNESS, AND WHAT IS TYPICAL FOR EACH CAUSE? (CONTINUED)

CAUSE	WHAT IS IT?	TYPICAL SYMPTOMS
Severe systemic infection	Severe body-wide infection, caused by bacteria in the blood	History of cough, painful or difficult urination, abdominal pain, fever, shaking chills
Brain abscess	A collection of pus resulting from an infection in the brain	Persistent headache, fever, sometimes stiff neck
Diabetic ketoacidosis	A complication of untreated diabetes	Recent fever, vomiting, rapid breathing, sweet-smelling breath, overproduction of urine, gradual lapse into coma
Respiratory failure	Failure of the lungs	Shallow or slow breathing, recent lung infection, gradual lapse into coma; occurs more commonly in people with a history of chronic lung disease
Chronic renal failure	Inability of the kidneys to function properly	Pallor, gradual lapse into coma, history of kidney disease
Acute renal failure	Sudden loss of function in the kidneys, often associated with medications	Decreased urine output, blood in urine, nausea, drowsiness, trouble breathing
Intracranial hemorrhage	Bleeding in or around the brain	Sudden and severe headache, nausea, vomiting, fever, stiff neck, rapid loss of consciousness
Hypertensive encephalopathy	Brain disease caused by chronic high blood pressure	History of high blood pressure, confusion, may occur in the last months of pregnancy

CAUSE	WHAT IS IT?	TYPICAL SYMPTOMS
Cerebral infarction	Stroke	Loss of consciousness can occur rapidly or gradually, more common in the elderly and people with a history of diabetes, high blood pressure, stroke, or heart attack
Brain tumor	Unchecked, abnormal growth of cells in the brain	Chronic and persistent headache, nausea, vomiting, coma
Shock	Body-wide shutdown	Cold and clammy skin, sometimes recent history of infection or severe bleeding from an injury
Feigned coma	Faking a coma	History of emotional problems

WHAT CAN CAUSE LOSS OF CONSCIOUSNESS, AND WHAT IS TYPICAL FOR EACH CAUSE? (CONTINUED)

Other causes of coma include having too much sodium or calcium in the blood, thyroid or pituitary problems, acid imbalance, or liver failure.

Menstrual Cramps

What it feels like: waves of pain and aching in the lower back, abdomen, and thighs that disappear when you begin menstruating each month.

Your Doctor Visit

What your doctor will ask you about: depression, anxiety, irritability, decreased interest in usual activities, difficulty concentrating, lethargy, change in appetite, change in sleep patterns, breast tenderness, bloating, weight gain. The doctor will also want to know if you have ever had an ultrasound of the vagina or a biopsy of your cervix, and what those examinations showed, or if you have taken nonsteroidal anti-inflammatory medications such as ibuprofen, or if you have taken soy or other herbal remedies.

Your doctor will do a physical examination including a thorough rectal and pelvic exam.

WHAT ARE THE DIFFERENT TYPES OF MENSTRUAL CRAMPS, AND WHAT IS TYPICAL FOR EACH TYPE?		
TYPE	WHAT IS IT?	TYPICAL SYMPTOMS
Dysmenorrhea	Painful menstrual periods	Several days of pain in the lower back, abdomen, and thighs, pain disappears when menstruation begins
Premenstrual dysphoric syndrome	A more severe form of what is commonly known as premenstrual syndrome (PMS)	To have premenstrual dysphoric syndrome, you must have at least five of the following symptoms: depression, anxiety, irritability, decreased interest in usual activities, difficulty concentrating, fatigue and weakness, changes in appetite, changes in sleeping patterns, breast tenderness, bloating, or weight gain
Endometriosis	Overgrowth of tissue from the uterus	Constant pain, increasing in severity until menstrual flow becomes light

Mental Delays (Child)

What it feels like: the child does not exhibit mental skills seen in children of similar ages; also known as mental retardation.

What can make it worse: asking the child to look at or listen to something, emotional upset.

Not every healthy child develops at the same pace, and it is difficult to determine if a child is mentally developing normally during the first few months of life. Most children who initially appear to be "slow starters" eventually catch up to their peers.

Your Doctor Visit

What your doctor will ask about the child: abnormal hearing, trouble seeing, difficult behavior, convulsions, disturbances in sensation or movement, results of tests of reading, vision, and hearing.

Your doctor will want to know if the child or anyone in the child's family has had any of these conditions: prematurity, convulsions at birth, deformities, low Apgar score, jaundice.

Your doctor may also ask if the child's mother experienced any of the following conditions during pregnancy: rash, lymph node enlargement, German measles, unusually long or short labor, prolonged anesthesia, blood infections.

Your doctor will want to know when the child first began to appear "delayed," and the nature of the delays.

Your doctor will ask you if the child has been eating lead paint or dirt, and the nature of the child's family life.

Your doctor will want to know if the child is taking any medications.

Your doctor will do a physical examination including the following: checking for the presence of certain development milestones, measuring head circumference, height, weight, checking ears, thorough eye exam, pushing on the abdomen.

Important factors to consider when visiting a doctor to ask about a child's mental delays:

- The only person who should diagnose a child with mental retardation is an expert in **developmental neurology**.

- Before diagnosing a child as mentally retarded, your doctor will conduct **a number of tests** of different aspects of mental function **at regular intervals**.

- Most cases of mental retardation involve delays in one area of mental function. Multiple types of delays in one child may be the result of environmental problems, such as child abuse, neglect, or changes in school. Certain diseases can also produce multiple delays, including muscle disease, poor vision, and nervous system disease.

- The following factors are associated with a higher risk of mental delays in children:

  - **Rubella** during the first 12 weeks or **blood infections** during any stage of the mother's pregnancy

  - Being born with **yellowing skin** (see chapter on Yellow Skin; this condition is often normal)**, seizures, a low Apgar score** (the number given by the doctor when the baby is born that tells how well she is breathing and how well her heart is beating)**, cerebral palsy, Down syndrome, prematurity**

  - **Infantile hypothyroidism**, in which the infant's thyroid gland is not sufficiently active; symptoms of hypothyroidism in an infant include increasing weight relative to height, yellow skin, thick tongue, and slow development

Mouth Trouble

What it feels like: varies from pain to bleeding to trouble swallowing.

Your Doctor Visit

What your doctor will ask you about: growths in the mouth, foul-smelling breath, sore or bleeding gums, recent skin abnormalities, common cold, difficulty talking, difficulty swallowing, sounds heard while breathing, excessive alcohol drinking, toothache, facial pain, salivation problems, fever, unpleasant taste.

Your doctor will want to know if you or anyone in your family has had any of these conditions: diabetes, syphilis, alcoholism, human immunodeficiency virus (HIV).

Your doctor will want to know if you smoke, wear dentures, brush and floss your teeth regularly, and if you have recently come in contact with a person who has strep throat.

Your doctor will want to know if you're taking any of these medications: diphenylhydantoin (Dilantin), antibiotics, steroids.

Your doctor will do a physical examination including the following: temperature, mouth exam, throat exam, checking lymph nodes for swelling.

WHAT CAN CAUSE MOUTH TROUBLE, AND WHAT IS TYPICAL FOR EACH CAUSE?

INFECTIONS OF THE MOUTH, THROAT, LIPS, AND GUMS

CAUSE	WHAT IS IT?	TYPICAL SYMPTOMS
Pharyngitis	Sore throat, caused by a viral or bacterial infection	Recent contact with another person with a sore throat, malaise, earache, runny nose, fever
Canker sore	Painful ulcer in the mouth or on the lips	Painful sore, sometimes fever and swollen lymph nodes
Candidiasis	Yeast infection that occurs more commonly in diabetics, infants, people with HIV, and those taking antibiotics or steroids	White, creamy lesions in the mouth, soreness, bleeding gums, unpleasant taste
"Trench mouth"	Progressive mouth disease	History of poor oral hygiene, foul-smelling breath, bleeding gums
Mononucleosis	Viral infection known as "mono"	Sore throat, fatigue, swollen lymph nodes in the neck
Herpangina	Disease marked by sudden sore throat	Sudden sore throat, fever, occurs more commonly in children
Gingivostomatitis	Inflammation in the gums and mouth	Sore mouth, fever, ulcers on the tongue and gums
Peritonsillar abscess	Collection of pus around the tonsils	Severe pain, trouble talking and swallowing, fever, occurs more commonly in children
Epiglottitis	Inflammation of the throat structure that blocks air passages	Vibrating sound when breathing, muffled speaking, sore throat, trouble swallowing, drooling, occurs more commonly in children aged 3 to 7 years

WHAT CAN CAUSE MOUTH TROUBLE, AND WHAT IS TYPICAL FOR EACH CAUSE? (CONTINUED)

GUM DISEASE

CAUSE	WHAT IS IT?	TYPICAL SYMPTOMS
Gingival hypertrophy	Swelling in the gums	Gum swelling, occurs in people taking diphenylhydantoin (Dilantin)
Periodontal disease	A disease of the tissue that supports teeth	Sore and bleeding gums, tooth plaque, gum swelling, recession of gums to expose roots of teeth, history of poor dental hygiene

LIP DISEASE

CAUSE	WHAT IS IT?	TYPICAL SYMPTOMS
Herpes simplex	Disease caused by the herpes virus that produces watery blisters around the mouth and lips	Painful blisters on lips or in mouth, may recur
Cheilosis	Condition in which the lips become scaly	Chronic cracking and inflammation at the corner of the mouth, occurs in people without teeth

GROWTHS AROUND THE MOUTH, LIPS, AND GUMS

CAUSE	WHAT IS IT?	TYPICAL SYMPTOMS
Leukoplakia	Formation of thick, white patches of tissue inside the mouth	Painless white patches of tissue inside the mouth, not removable with cotton swab, history of cigarette smoking
Neoplasia	Abnormal, unchecked growth of cells	Lumps, persistent sores, pain, bleeding gums, unpleasant taste

WHAT CAN CAUSE MOUTH TROUBLE, AND WHAT IS TYPICAL FOR EACH CAUSE? (CONTINUED)

TOOTHACHE

CAUSE	WHAT IS IT?	TYPICAL SYMPTOMS
Dental cavity	Disease that affects tooth structure	Initial pain only with hot or cold food, facial pain, eventually pain becomes constant
Sinusitis	Inflammation and infection of spaces in the bones of the face	Facial pain that increases when bending over, runny nose, fever

Muscle Weakness

What it feels like: muscular fatigue, causing problems getting around and performing day-to-day activities.

If your muscles feel strong but you feel weak, see the chapter on Weakness for more information. If your muscle weakness has occurred suddenly, see the chapter on Numbness, Loss of Movement, and Trouble Talking to make sure you are not experiencing a stroke.

Your Doctor Visit

What your doctor will ask you about: neck pain, back pain, muscle pain, muscle twitching, blurred or double vision, changes in sensation or speech, heat intolerance, obesity, abnormal hair growth.

Your doctor will want to know if you or anyone in your family has had any of these conditions: chronic disease, alcoholism, disease of the discs in the back, nervous system disease, thyroid disease, muscle weakness.

Your doctor will want to know if the weakness occurs all over, or in particular regions of the body, and if it occurs sporadically or has worsened with time.

Your doctor will want to know if you're taking any of these medications: steroids, statins to treat high cholesterol.

Your doctor will ask you if you have been exposed to insecticides or received a vaccine against polio, and if you feel particularly weak when arising from a chair.

Your doctor will do a physical examination including tests of reflexes, movement, and sensation.

WHAT CAN CAUSE MUSCLE WEAKNESS, AND WHAT IS TYPICAL FOR EACH CAUSE?		
CAUSE	WHAT IS IT?	TYPICAL SYMPTOMS
Muscular dystrophy	Hereditary disease characterized by progressive muscle wasting	Progressive weakness, difficulty getting up from a chair, family history of dystrophy
Myositis	Infection that causes pain or weakness in muscles	Weakness, pain, tenderness
Disuse atrophy	Wasting of muscles after long disuse, perhaps following disease	Occurs in people with disabling illness, such as stroke or arthritis
Drug use	Weakness caused by certain medications	Occurs in people taking steroids, statins, and diuretics ("water pills"), and in heavy alcohol drinkers
Endocrine disease	Disease affecting the hormones	Heat intolerance, weight gain in the abdomen, abnormal hair growth
Insecticide poisoning	Ingesting a toxic amount of insecticides	Double vision, weakness of speech, weakness worsens at the end of the day, fatigue after exercise
Peripheral neuropathy	Disease of the nerves in the extremities that occurs more commonly in people who drink heavily or have diabetes	Weakness occurs in one body region, change in sensation
Nervous system disease	Abnormalities in the brain or spinal cord	Regional weakness, abnormal sensation
Guillain-Barré syndrome	Disease characterized by inflammation in the nerves	Weakness and paralysis that begins in the legs, may progress rapidly
Poliomyelitis	Disease caused by the polio virus that can lead to paralysis	Fever, rapid onset of widespread weakness, no history of immunization against the virus

CAUSE	WHAT IS IT?	TYPICAL SYMPTOMS
WHAT CAN CAUSE MUSCLE WEAKNESS, AND WHAT IS TYPICAL FOR EACH CAUSE?		
Amyotrophic lateral sclerosis	Disease of the nerve cells that can lead to loss of control over movements, also known as Lou Gehrig disease	Slowly progressive weakness, occurs only in adults
Werdnig-Hoffman disease	Genetic disease that can lead to progressive muscle weakness	Generalized weakness, lack of reflexes, occurs only in children

Nail Problems

What it feels like: varies from pain to swelling and redness to discoloration.

What can make it worse: injury, constant immersion in water, contact with chemicals, nail biting.

Your Doctor Visit

What your doctor will ask you about: pain, swelling, redness, discoloration, pitting or nail destruction, any adjacent abnormalities in the skin.

Your doctor will want to know if you or anyone in your family has had any of these conditions: chronic lung disease, chronic heart disease, thyroid disease, diabetes, psoriasis, nail problems.

Your doctor will want to know if you have been exposed to chemicals or have spent a lot of time with your hands underwater.

Your doctor will want to know if you're taking any medications.

Your doctor will do a physical examination including a thorough examination of your fingers, nails, and the surrounding tissue.

WHAT CAN CAUSE VARIOUS NAIL PROBLEMS, AND WHAT IS TYPICAL FOR EACH CAUSE?

COMMON NAIL PROBLEMS

CAUSE	WHAT IS IT?	TYPICAL SYMPTOMS
Warts (See chapter on Skin Problems.)	Painless growth on fingers	Painless gray-brown or flesh-colored growth, occurs more commonly in adolescents
Separation of nails from fingertips	Nail separates from the skin of the fingertip	Often occurs after injury, may occur as a result of thyroid disease
Infection	Invasion of the nail by bacteria or yeast	Inflammation of the skin under the nail, redness, swelling of surrounding skin, often occurs after constant immersion in water or injury, more common in diabetics
Clubbing	Distortions in finger nails, often the result of diseases that restrict oxygen flow to fingers	Deformity in the fingertip, history of heart disease or chronic lung disease

NAIL PAIN

CAUSE	WHAT IS IT?	TYPICAL SYMPTOMS
Hematoma	A mass that forms after a blood vessel breaks	Blue-black discoloration under the nail, usually occurs after injury
Glomus tumor	Benign growth of cells under the nail	Severe and recurrent pain, pink growth under nail, sometimes occurs after injury

WHAT CAN CAUSE VARIOUS NAIL PROBLEMS, AND WHAT IS TYPICAL FOR EACH CAUSE? (CONTINUED)

NAIL DESTRUCTION

CAUSE	WHAT IS IT?	TYPICAL SYMPTOMS
Nail biting	Habit of biting off nails	History of nail biting
Fungus infection	Invasion of the nail by a fungus	Often occurs after constant immersion in water
Psoriasis	Skin disease marked by red patches and white scaly areas	History of scaly skin patches on arms and legs

Nausea and Vomiting (Adult)

What it feels like: Feeling sick to your stomach and throwing up.

What can make it worse: pregnancy, eating contaminated food, drinking too much alcohol, motion sickness, having recently stopped taking steroids.

In general, vomiting blood is more serious than just vomiting.

Your Doctor Visit

What your doctor will ask you about: fever, feeling as if the room is spinning, ear ringing, headache, change in movement or mental function, excessive thirst, chest pain, diarrhea, abdominal pain or swelling, black or bloody bowel movements, vomiting blood, light stools, dark urine, yellowing skin, red spots on skin, skin bruising, muscle aches, weakness, results of tests of gastrointestinal function, previous blood transfusions.

Your doctor will want to know if you or anyone in your family has had any of these conditions: blood vessel problems in the esophagus (the tube connecting the back of the throat to the stomach), ulcer disease, gastritis, liver disease, alcoholism, blood disease, bleeding disorder, gastrointestinal bleeding, diabetes, cardiovascular disease, pregnancy.

Your doctor will want to know what you have been throwing up, and how much you have thrown up.

Your doctor will also ask if you have been in recent contact with people suffering from nausea and vomiting or the liver disease hepatitis (see below).

**If you are vomiting blood, your doctor will want to know how
many times this has occurred, how much blood you are throwing
up, and whether the blood appears bright red or darker brown.**

**Your doctor will want to know if you're taking any medications,
including:** aspirin, warfarin (Coumadin), the painkiller indomethacin
(Indocin), alcohol, steroids.

**Your doctor will do a physical examination including the fol-
lowing:** blood pressure, temperature, pulse, thorough eye exam,
checking the throat, pushing on the abdomen, checking stool for the
presence of blood, testing your memory, thorough skin exam.

WHAT CAN CAUSE NAUSEA AND VOMITING IN ADULTS, AND WHAT IS TYPICAL FOR EACH CAUSE?

NAUSEA AND VOMITING IN GENERAL

CAUSE	WHAT IS IT?	TYPICAL SYMPTOMS
Pregnancy	Nausea and vomiting that occur early in pregnancy, also known as "morning sickness"	Lack of menstrual period
Chronic indigestion	Trouble digesting food	Chronic nausea, no vomiting
Acute gastroenteritis (See chapters on Diarrhea and Abdominal Pain.)	Infection of the stomach	Diarrhea, abdominal pain, muscle aches, mild fever, may occur after eating contaminated food
Acute hepatitis	Liver infection	Diarrhea, abdominal pain, muscle aches, mild fever, light stools, dark urine, yellowing skin, occurs after contact with people infected with hepatitis
Medications, chemicals, alcohol	Taking too much of a medication, chemical, or alcohol	Otherwise normal

**WHAT CAN CAUSE NAUSEA AND VOMITING IN ADULTS,
AND WHAT IS TYPICAL FOR EACH CAUSE? (CONTINUED)**

NAUSEA AND VOMITING IN GENERAL

CAUSE	WHAT IS IT?	TYPICAL SYMPTOMS
Labyrinthine disorders (See chapter on Dizziness.)	Inner ear problems	Vertigo, ringing in the ears, motion sickness
Diabetic acidosis	Buildup of substances in the blood as a result of diabetes	History of diabetes, loss of appetite, excessive thirst, excessive secretion of urine
Adrenal insufficiency	Lack of hormones made by the adrenal gland that can result from suddenly quitting caffeine	Abdominal pain, irritability, tiredness, occasional fever, often occurs after abrupt cessation of steroids
Brain swelling	Swelling of the brain or its coverings	Headache, changes in muscle strength or mental function
Myocardial infarction	Heart attack	Chest pain, sweating, history of heart disease

VOMITING BLOOD

CAUSE	WHAT IS IT?	TYPICAL SYMPTOMS
Peptic ulcer	Severe irritation of the stomach or intestinal lining	Burning upper abdominal pain that is worse when lying down, sometimes relieved by food or antacids and made worse by aspirin, drugs such as ibuprofen, or alcohol
Gastritis	Serious irritation of the stomach	Often painless, can occur after taking too much aspirin or drinking too much alcohol

**WHAT CAN CAUSE NAUSEA AND VOMITING IN ADULTS,
AND WHAT IS TYPICAL FOR EACH CAUSE? (CONTINUED)**

VOMITING BLOOD

CAUSE	WHAT IS IT?	TYPICAL SYMPTOMS
Esophageal varices	Blood vessel problems associated with the esophagus, which connects the back of the throat to the stomach, that occur most often in people who drink heavily	Yellowing of the skin
Esophageal tear	Tear in the esophagus resulting from prolonged vomiting	History of long bouts of retching before vomiting blood
Bleeding disorders	Problems with bleeding, such as trouble clotting	Family history of bleeding easily or excessively

Nausea and Vomiting (Child)

What it feels like: feeling sick to your stomach and throwing up.

What can make it worse: feeling scared or excited, eating certain foods, ingesting drugs or poison, head injury.

What can make it better: burping.

Your Doctor Visit

What your doctor will ask about: fever, weight loss, headache, earache, sore throat, vomiting blood, abdominal swelling or pain, diarrhea, decrease in bowel movements, crying on urination, dark urine, weakness, dizziness when standing, skin bruising, red spots on skin, yellowing skin, blood in stool.

Your doctor will want to know if the child or anyone in the child's family has had any of these conditions: blood vessel problems in the esophagus (the tube connecting the back of the throat to the stomach), ulcer disease, gastritis, liver disease, bleeding disorders, gastrointestinal bleeding.

Your doctor will want to know what the child has been throwing up, and how much the child has thrown up.

Your doctor will also ask if the child has been in recent contact with people suffering from nausea and vomiting or the liver disease hepatitis (see below).

If the child is vomiting blood, your doctor will want to know how many times this has occurred, how much blood the child is throwing up, and whether the blood appears bright red or darker brown.

Your doctor will want to know if the child is taking any medications, including: aspirin, indomethacin (Indocin), steroids.

Your doctor will do a physical examination including the following: pulse, weight, height, thorough eye exam, checking the neck for stiffness, looking in the throat, pushing on the abdomen, checking stool for the presence of blood, thorough skin exam.

WHAT CAN CAUSE NAUSEA AND VOMITING IN CHILDREN, AND WHAT IS TYPICAL FOR EACH CAUSE?

NAUSEA AND VOMITING IN GENERAL

CAUSE	WHAT IS IT?	TYPICAL SYMPTOMS
Gastroesophageal reflux	The movement of stomach acid up into and through the esophagus, which connects the throat to the stomach	Often relieved by frequent burping or changing feeding schedule, occurs more commonly in premature infants
Acute gastroenteritis (See chapter on Abdominal Pain.)	Infection of the stomach	Diarrhea, abdominal pain, muscle aches, mild fever
Systemic infection	Body-wide infection, perhaps resulting from ear infection, tonsillitis, or a kidney infection	Fever, severe vomiting, diarrhea
Hepatitis	Liver infection	Diarrhea, abdominal pain, muscle aches, mild fever, light stools, dark urine, yellowing skin, occurs after contact with people infected with hepatitis
High bowel obstruction	Blockage in the upper bowel	Persistent vomiting, a large amount of food in vomit, may vomit blood, weight loss, usually occurs in first three months of life
Lower bowel obstruction	Blockage in the lower bowel	Green bile in vomit, decrease or lack of bowel movements, occurs in children younger than 2 years

WHAT CAN CAUSE NAUSEA AND VOMITING IN CHILDREN, AND WHAT IS TYPICAL FOR EACH CAUSE? (CONTINUED)

NAUSEA AND VOMITING IN GENERAL

CAUSE	WHAT IS IT?	TYPICAL SYMPTOMS
Brain injury	Occurs as a result of inflammation, tumor, or injury in the brain	Head holding, headache, tiredness, projectile vomiting
Poison or medications	Ingestion of poison or too much of a medication	Behavioral changes, unconsciousness
Metabolic disease	Disease affecting the way food and other substances are broken down	Vomiting soon after birth, vomiting after trying a food for the first time, weight loss
Psychologic disturbance	Vomiting following fright or excitement, or in order to get attention	Otherwise normal

VOMITING BLOOD

CAUSE	WHAT IS IT?	TYPICAL SYMPTOMS
Esophageal tear	Tear in the tissue of the tube that connects the back of the throat to the stomach	History of long bouts of retching before vomiting blood
Bleeding disorders	Problems with bleeding, such as trouble clotting	Family history of bleeding easily or excessively

It is very rare for a child to vomit blood. The most common reasons for blood appearing in vomit are ingesting blood from the nose and mouth, during childbirth, or from a bleeding nipple.

Neck Problems

What it feels like: varies from pain to tightness to swelling or tenderness in the neck, sometimes with difficulty moving the neck.

What can make it worse: raising your arms over your head, stretching your neck far in any direction.

If your pain stems from lumps in your neck, refer to the chapter on Swelling for more information. If your pain began after an injury, see the chapter on Injury for more information.

Your Doctor Visit

What your doctor will ask you about: headache, change in strength or feeling, fever, chills, swelling in the neck, tenderness in the neck, shoulder pain, chest pain, nausea, vomiting.

Your doctor will want to know if you or anyone in your family has had any of these conditions: heart disease, any nervous system disease, arthritis, cancer.

Your doctor will want to know if your neck pain began after an injury or a car accident.

Your doctor will want to know if you're taking any medications, including antipsychotic medications, including phenothiazines, such as haloperidol (Haldol).

Your doctor will do a physical examination including the following: temperature, checking your neck for tenderness and range of motion, testing reflexes and strength and feeling in the arms and legs, a series of experiments to determine the cause of your neck pain.

WHAT CAN CAUSE NECK PROBLEMS, AND WHAT IS TYPICAL FOR EACH CAUSE?		
CAUSE	WHAT IS IT?	TYPICAL SYMPTOMS
Referred pain to the neck	Pain radiating to the neck from the chest, perhaps a result of heart disease	History of angina or heart attack, occurs only in adults (See chapter on Chest Pain.)
Muscle strain	Injury to the muscles of the neck	Dull ache in the back of the neck, tenderness, muscle spasm, history of injury or strain; may occur after whiplash injury from a car accident
Cervical disk disease	A disorder affecting the vertebrae of the neck	Headache focused on the back of the head, decreased range of neck motion, sometimes weakness in arms or legs, numbness or shooting pain in shoulders, arms, or hands
Arthritis	Joint inflammation in the bones of the neck	Headache focused on the back of the head, decreased range of neck motion, sometimes weakness in arms or legs, numbness or shooting pain in shoulders, arms, or hands (See chapter on Joint Pain.)
Infection	Inflammation and pain caused by a pathogen	Persistent pain in the back of the neck, pain may be severe
Meningismus	Irritation of the covering of the brain	Aching and stiff neck, headache, fever, nausea, vomiting
Dystonic reaction	Problems in the neck muscles	Painful and involuntary spasms in muscles of neck or jaw, occurs in people who recently began taking phenothiazines such as Haldol

Numbness, Loss of Movement, or Trouble Talking

What it feels like: can include a loss of feeling, dull pain, or a sensation of "pins and needles" in certain parts of your body, blurred vision, loss of balance, trouble speaking or swallowing, loss of consciousness, headache, stiff neck.

What can make it worse: injury, feeling cold, placing strong pressure on areas close to the numb region.

If you are feeling numbness accompanied by other symptoms such as headache, blurred vision, and loss of speech, you may be experiencing a stroke, and should seek medical attention immediately.

Your Doctor Visit

What your doctor will ask you about: headache, anxiety, depression, numbness in hands or around mouth, weakness, muscle wasting or tenderness, lack of coordination, change in vision or hearing, change in speech, neck pain, back pain.

Your doctor will want to know if you or anyone in your family has had any of these conditions: any nervous system disease, cardiovascular disease, diabetes, high blood pressure, emotional problems, alcoholism, anemia, syphilis, cancer, kidney disease.

Your doctor will want to know if you have other feelings besides numbness, if you feel numb constantly or intermittently, and where exactly you feel numb.

If you are also having trouble talking, your doctor may ask you questions to ensure you are not having a stroke. For instance, your doctor may ask if you are experiencing a stiff neck, blurred vision, convulsions, or a loss of consciousness.

Your doctor will want to know if you're taking any medications, including: isoniazid, nitrofurantoin (Furadantin), warfarin (Coumadin), heart medications, birth control pills, drugs to control high blood pressure.

Your doctor will want to know if you have recently been exposed to arsenic or large amounts of lead.

Your doctor will do a physical examination including the following: blood pressure, pulse, tests of reflexes, balance, coordination, and sensation.

Most commonly, numbness results from conditions that can also cause pain in joints, legs, arms, hands, and feet. See chapters on those symptoms for more information, or the table below for less common causes of numbness.

WHAT CAN CAUSE NUMBNESS, LOSS OF MOVEMENT, *AND TROUBLE TALKING, AND WHAT IS TYPICAL FOR EACH CAUSE?*		
CAUSE	**WHAT IS IT?**	**TYPICAL SYMPTOMS**
Hyper-ventilation	Breathing rapidly and deeply over an extended period	Numbness in both hands, faintness, pins and needles around lips, trouble breathing
Transient ischemic attack	A type of stroke in which there is a temporary halt in the flow of blood to part of the brain, lasts no longer than 24 hours	Numbness on one side of the body, clumsiness, trouble speaking, trouble seeing; occurs more commonly in the elderly and in people with diabetes, heart disease, or high blood pressure
Stroke	A failure of blood to get to the brain, either because of excessive bleeding in the brain causing a blockage or a clot in the blood vessels supplying the brain	Numbness on one side of the body, clumsiness, trouble speaking, trouble seeing; occurs more commonly in the elderly and in people with diabetes, cardiovascular disease, and high blood pressure; lasts longer than a transient ischemic attack

WHAT CAN CAUSE NUMBNESS, LOSS OF MOVEMENT, AND TROUBLE TALKING, AND WHAT IS TYPICAL FOR EACH CAUSE? (CONTINUED)

CAUSE	WHAT IS IT?	TYPICAL SYMPTOMS
Demyelinating disease	Disease involving the loss of the protective coating of nerves	Repeated episodes of numbness in various parts of the body
Peripheral neuropathy	Disease of the nerves in the body extremities	Weakness, occurs more commonly in alcoholics, diabetics, and people with kidney disease or anemia; may occur after exposure to certain drugs or toxic metals
Nerve compression	Compression of any of the nerves	Sharp pain or numbness in a particular region of an extremity, back or neck pain
Central nervous system damage	Disorders of the brain or spinal cord	Changes in sensation, strength, and coordination

Trouble talking in children —stammering, stuttering, and mispronunciation of sounds —is not uncommon, but does not mean there is an underlying brain problem. Hoarseness can be caused by infection or smoking (see chapter on Hoarseness).

Overdose or Poisoning

What it is: taking too much of a medication or ingesting a toxic substance.

If you believe that you or someone you know has ingested too much of a medication or a toxic substance, seek medical attention immediately by calling your local poison control center at 1-800-222-1222, before attempting to treat the problem yourself with syrup of ipecac or any other substance.

Your Doctor Visit

What your doctor will ask you about: loss of consciousness, hyperactivity, abnormal breathing, fever, low temperature, change in skin color, convulsions, tremors, spasms.

Your doctor will want to know if you or anyone in your family has had any of these conditions: previous overdose, poisoning, suicide attempts, depression, emotional problems, alcohol or drug abuse, any chronic disease.

Your doctor will want to know what you ingested and how much, and if you have been contemplating suicide.

Your doctor will want to know if you're taking any medications.

Your doctor will do a physical examination including the following: blood pressure, pulse, breathing rate, temperature, tests of mental alertness, looking inside the throat, listening to the chest with a stethoscope, pushing on the abdomen, thorough skin exam, checking sensation and reflexes.

If the patient is a child, the doctor will likely recommend that all potentially toxic substances be placed out of reach, to prevent future incidents.

The doctor may ask you to bring in samples of all the potential sources of the poisoning.

Depending on what substance was ingested, the doctor may try to get you to regurgitate it or rid the body of it in another way. **Do not attempt to do this yourself** before calling a poison control center at 1-800-222-1222, as the substances may cause more damage traveling back through your digestive system than they normally would.

If you have any questions about specific poisons, contact your **local poison control center** listed in the phone book.

Overeating

What it feels like: believing that you eat more than you should.

The amount of calories you need every day depends on your gender and size. Normal intake for moderately active men ranges from 2200 to 2800 calories per day, and for women ranges from 1800 to 2100 calories.

Your Doctor Visit

What your doctor will ask you about: anxiety, depression, eating to relieve stress, changes in weight, excessive urination, excessive thirst, ability to tolerate heat, weakness.

Your doctor will want to know if you or anyone in your family has had any of these conditions: diabetes, thyroid disease, emotional problems, obesity, recent cessation of smoking.

Your doctor will want to know why you think you eat too much, how much food you typically eat every day, and whether you engage in eating "binges."

Your doctor will want to know if you're taking any of these medications: antidepressants, antipsychotics, lithium.

Your doctor will do a physical examination including the following: weight, height, eye exam, thorough neck exam.

WHAT CAN CAUSE OVEREATING, AND WHAT IS TYPICAL FOR EACH CAUSE?		
CAUSE	**WHAT IS IT?**	**TYPICAL SYMPTOMS**
Smoking cessation	Recently giving up a smoking habit	Overeating
Hyper-thyroidism	Overactivity of the thyroid gland	Weight loss, hot flashes, sweating, sometimes a swollen gland in the neck
Diabetes	An inability to properly process sugar	Frequent drinking and urination, fatigue, sometimes double vision or weight loss
Medication use	Overeating as a result of taking antidepressants, antipsychotics, or lithium	Overeating because of a frequent feeling of hunger
Bulimia nervosa	Engaging in cycles of "binging" and "purging," in which you overeat and then starve yourself, vomit, or take laxatives	Binge eating followed by vomiting or taking laxatives
Parasitic infection of the intestines	Infection by tapeworm and other parasites	Overeating because of a frequent feeling of hunger

Poor Appetite

What it feels like: an inability to eat as much food as your body requires.

Your Doctor Visit

What your doctor will ask you about: weight loss, nausea, vomiting, fever, abdominal pain, jaundice (skin taking on a yellowish appearance), joint pains, bowel habits, changes in your emotional state, changes in sexual activity or sleep habits, your ability to concentrate.

Your doctor will want to know if you or anyone in your family has had any of these conditions: cancer, emotional problems, diseases affecting the kidneys or the circulatory or digestive systems.

If the patient is a child, your doctor will want to know if the child has any behavioral problems or plays with her food, how much she is expected to eat, and if she has a family history of cystic fibrosis.

Your doctor will want to know if you are taking any medications.

Your doctor will do a physical exam including the following: weight, height, temperature, listening to your chest and heart with a stethoscope, pushing on your abdomen, thorough skin examination, checking your limbs for swelling and muscular strength.

WHAT CAN CAUSE POOR APPETITE, AND WHAT IS TYPICAL FOR EACH CAUSE?

CAUSE	WHAT IS IT?	TYPICAL SYMPTOMS
Depression	A low mood that lasts for a series of days at a time	Feeling sad, difficulty sleeping and having sex, trouble concentrating
Anorexia nervosa	Fear of gaining weight	Dieting, excessive exercise, induced vomiting (in bulimia, also includes binge eating)
Cystic fibrosis (in children)	A genetic disease in which children become more prone to lung infections	Recurrent respiratory infections, coughing, weight loss
Gastroenteritis	Infection of the stomach and intestines	Nausea, vomiting, fever
Hepatitis	Infection or inflammation of the liver, due to alcoholism or viral infection	Nausea, vomiting, fever, jaundice (skin taking on a yellowish appearance)
Cancer	Unchecked, abnormal growth of cells	Varies depending on type of tumor; can include weakness
Crohn's disease	Chronic inflammation of the intestines	Bloody and/or frequent diarrhea, frequent abdominal pain
Parental anxiety (in children)	Parents may become anxious when children are too "fussy" in their eating habits	Usually weight is normal

Pregnancy

What it feels like: varies from nausea and vomiting to breast enlargement and weight gain.

Your Doctor Visit

What your doctor will ask you about: breast enlargement, nausea and vomiting, vaginal discharge or spotting, pelvic pressure or cramping, fetal "kicking," fever or chills, burning or frequent urination, ankle swelling, results of previous exams for this pregnancy.

Your doctor will want to know if you or anyone in your family has had any of these conditions: diabetes, hypertension, previous blood infections in pregnancy, sickle-cell disease, heart disease, rheumatic fever, drug addiction, previous uterine or pelvic surgery, previous cesarean delivery, kidney disease, thyroid disease, vaccination for rubella or history of rubella, genetic disease, Down syndrome, multiple births.

Your doctor will want to know the date of your last menstrual period and your age.

Your doctor may also ask you about your family life, and whether this pregnancy was planned.

Your doctor will want to know if you're taking any medications, particularly fertility drugs.

Your doctor will do a physical examination including the following: blood pressure, weight, pelvic exam, checking limbs for varicose veins or swelling, examining the position, size, and heart rate of the fetus.

Additional points to consider when visiting your doctor about pregnancy:

- Common **milestones** at different points in a pregnancy:

  - Week 16: The fetus begins to move, and your abdomen will likely be visibly larger.
  - Weeks 18 to 22: You can start to hear the fetus's heartbeat.

- During your doctor visit, you may be tested for **rubella and syphilis**, as well as **chlamydia and hepatitis B**.

- Your doctor will want to monitor your pregnancy particularly closely if any of the following are true:

  - You are younger than 18 or older than 35
  - You have a history of German measles or a skin rash with swollen lymph nodes in the first 12 weeks of pregnancy; you have a history of miscarriage; you were pregnant within the last 12 months; you have given birth to very tiny, very large, or premature babies; you have a history of multiple ectopic pregnancies (in which the fetus is implanted improperly)
  - You or your immediate family members have any of the diseases listed above at "Your doctor will want to know if you or anyone in your family has had any of these conditions"
  - You are obese, have high blood pressure, or have had an abnormal pelvic exam
  - Your pregnancy is unwanted or unplanned, or you have difficulties in your family or personal life

Sexual Problems and Inability to Conceive

What it feels like: not conceiving after 12 months of unprotected intercourse; or lack of interest in sex, lack of erection or ejaculation, premature ejaculation (men); or lack of interest in sex, pain with intercourse, lack of orgasm (women).

On average, fewer than 10 percent of women under the age of 35 fail to conceive after 12 months of unprotected intercourse. After 35, the rate of infertility among women increases.

Your Doctor Visit

What your doctor will ask you about: failure of erection, testicular pain or swelling, vaginal discharge, abdominal or pelvic pain, pain on intercourse, irregular periods, genital lesions, genital discharge, genital pain, back pain, calf or buttock pain caused by exercise, anxiety, depression, change in sleep pattern, appetite, change in bowel or bladder function, spontaneous erections, sexually transmitted diseases, results of previous semen analysis, pelvic examinations, baseline temperature, or pelvic endoscopy.

Your doctor will want to know if you or anyone in your family has had any of these conditions: abdominal surgery, pelvic surgery, emotional problems, mumps, endometriosis, past pregnancy or abortion, sexually transmitted disease, heart disease, diabetes, high blood pressure, infertility or sterility, prostate cancer, any recent surgery, nervous system disease, history of sexual assault.

If you are experiencing sexual problems, your doctor will want to know if the problem began recently, or has occurred for a long time. Your doctor may also ask you if you are currently experiencing job or family problems, and whose idea it was to seek help—yours or your partner's.

Your doctor will want to know if you're taking any of these medications: blood pressure pills, the antipsychotic Mellaril (thioridazine), antidepressants, hormone treatments, the diuretic ("water pill") spironolactone.

Your doctor will do a physical examination including the following: pulse, distribution of body hair, looking for skin lesions.

Men: checking size and consistency of testes and the opening of the penis, checking reflexes, sperm analysis.

Women: pelvic exam, checking the genital mucosa, looking for vaginal narrowing, checking for clitoral adhesions, basal temperature.

WHAT CAN CAUSE AN INABILITY TO CONCEIVE?	
CAUSE	**WHAT IS IT?**
Sperm problems	Few or poor-quality sperm
Inadequate ovulation	Inability to position an egg in the right place to be fertilized
Reproductive organ problems	Problems with the fallopian tubes, cervix, or uterus

WHAT CAN CAUSE SEXUAL PROBLEMS, AND WHAT IS TYPICAL FOR EACH CAUSE?		
CAUSE	**WHAT IS IT?**	**TYPICAL SYMPTOMS**
Emotional problems	Stress, difficulty coping with life changes, other mental problems	Troubled partner relationship, men can achieve erection but are unable to sustain it while intimate, women either fail to reach orgasm or experience pain during intercourse
Medication use	Blood pressure medications, antidepressants, the diuretic ("water pill") spironolactone, some antipsychotic drugs such as Mellaril (thioridazine)	Inability to achieve erection or orgasm

WHAT CAN CAUSE SEXUAL PROBLEMS, AND WHAT IS TYPICAL FOR EACH CAUSE? (CONTINUED)		
CAUSE	WHAT IS IT?	TYPICAL SYMPTOMS
Genital abnormalities (See chapter on Sexually Transmitted Diseases [STDs].)	Problems with the genitals	Pain on intercourse, lack of sensation, inability to achieve erection or ejaculate
Neurologic causes	Problems with the nervous system, uncommon	Lack of spontaneous erections, loss of bowel or bladder control
Hormonal causes	An imbalance of hormones in the body	Abnormal distribution of pubic hair
Chronic disease	Any long-term disease	Problems with sexual interest or functioning, sometimes associated with depression

Sexually Transmitted Diseases (STDs)

What it feels like: varies from discharge from the penis or vagina to genital sores to pelvic pain.

Not all instances of discharge from the penis or vagina are due to STDs; see below for more information.

If you are having sexual problems you believe are not caused by an STD, see the chapter on Sexual Problems and Inability to Conceive for more information.

Having certain STDs may mean that you are at risk for infection with HIV, the virus that causes AIDS, so your doctor may ask about other symptoms.

Your Doctor Visit

What your doctor will ask you about: swollen lymph nodes, pain with or difficulty urinating, genital sores, pelvic pain, fever, chills, eye inflammation, joint pain, recent skin rash, results of past tests for syphilis or HIV, the color of any discharge from the penis or vagina.

Your doctor will want to know if you or anyone in your family has had any of these conditions: syphilis, gonorrhea, pelvic inflammatory disease, allergy to penicillin or ampicillin.

Your doctor will want to know why you think you have an STD.

Your doctor may ask if you have oral, genital, or anal sex; if you or any of your sexual partners use IV drugs; if any of your partners have an STD; and whether you or your sexual partners have had many sexual partners.

Your doctor will do a physical examination including the following: pelvic exam, taking culture of the cervix, testing discharge from the penis. If the penis initially produces no discharge, your doctor may perform a rectal exam and massage the prostate to obtain a discharge.

WHAT ARE SOME STDs, AND WHAT IS TYPICAL FOR EACH?

CAUSE	WHAT IS IT?	TYPICAL SYMPTOMS
Chlamydia	Bacterial infection	Watery vaginal discharge, bleeding after sex, infertility if left untreated
Herpes	Recurrent genital sores caused by infection with a virus	Painful genital sores, watery discharge, painful urination
Syphilis	Bacterial infection	Painless genital ulcer, rash
Gonorrhea	Bacterial infection	Abdominal pain, fever, chills, green or yellow discharge
Chancroid	Bacterial infection	Painful genital ulcer, swelling in the groin
Trichomonas urethritis	Parasitic infection	Itching around the urethra, painful urination, thick and clear discharge from the penis, vaginal itching and smelly discharge

DISCHARGE UNRELATED TO STDs (MALE)

CAUSE	WHAT IS IT?	TYPICAL SYMPTOMS
Urethritis	Inflammation of the urethra, the tube that drains urine from the bladder	Clear and watery discharge, pain with urination
Reiter's syndrome	Disease triggered by an infection, in which men develop a recurrence of urethritis (see above)	Painful urination, frequent and persistent thick penile discharge, joint pain, eye inflammation, more common in young men

Shakiness

What it feels like: involuntary rhythmic or non-rhythmic body movements.

What can make it worse: rest, movement, anxiety, alcohol, falling asleep, fatigue.

Your doctor may distinguish between different forms of shakiness. For instance, rhythmic, involuntary movements in the arms and legs are often called *tremors*, while doctors often refer to sudden, jerking, and nonrhythmic body movements as *twitches*.

Your Doctor Visit

What your doctor will ask you about: muscle weakness, recent joint pain, fever, skin rash, convulsions, anxiety, depression, strange feelings, abnormal strength or sensations, lack of equilibrium, change in writing, yellowing of skin, results of previous tests of brain function.

Your doctor will want to know if you or anyone in your family has had any of these conditions: alcoholism, delirium tremens, emotional problems, liver disease, nervous system disease, Parkinson's disease, thyroid disease, drug addiction, syphilis, rheumatic fever, birth injury, mental retardation, similar shakiness.

Your doctor will want to know when you first began to notice your shakiness, and what areas of your body are involved.

Your doctor will want to know if you're taking any of these medications: alcohol, diphenylhydantoin (Dilantin), L-dopa, benzotropine (Cogentin), metoclopramide (Reglan), tranquilizers, lithium (Eskalith), antidepressants, phenothiazines such as chlorpromazine (Thorazine) or haloperidol (Haldol).

In rare instances, people may develop a twitching in the body after exposure to insecticides.

Your doctor will do a physical examination including the following: pulse, temperature, checking neck for enlargement of the thyroid, pushing on the abdomen, checking for rigidity, listening to the heart with a stethoscope, testing for movement, strength, reflexes, facial expressions, and balance.

Your doctor may also ask you to try to suppress the shakiness.

WHAT CAN CAUSE TREMORS, AND WHAT IS TYPICAL FOR EACH CAUSE?		
CAUSE	WHAT IS IT?	TYPICAL SYMPTOMS
Anxiety	Feeling anxious	Tremors present during movement or when holding one position, sweaty palms, history of severe or chronic emotional stress
Drug withdrawal	Painful symptoms that occur when coming off of an addictive substance	Tremors present during movement or when holding one position, fever, delirium, history of drug addiction
Inherited tremor	Tremor passed down through families, also known as "essential tremor"	Tremors present during movement or when holding one position, family history of tremor, develops later in life, may disappear when drinking alcohol or taking beta-blockers
Hyperthyroidism	Overactivity of the thyroid gland	Tremors present during movement or when holding one position, weight loss despite good appetite, inability to tolerate heat
Medication use	Tremor induced by certain medications	Tremors present during movement or when holding one position, follows use of lithium or antidepressants

WHAT CAN CAUSE TREMORS, AND WHAT IS TYPICAL FOR EACH CAUSE? (CONTINUED)		
CAUSE	WHAT IS IT?	TYPICAL SYMPTOMS
Parkinson's disease	Nervous system disease that produces tremors	Tremors present at rest and disappear with movement, shuffling, use of metoclopramide (Reglan)
Other nervous system diseases	Certain nervous system diseases which produce tremors that increase with particular movements	No tremors at rest, tremors increase with particular movements such as finger-to-nose testing, history of neurologic disease, lack of coordination, unsteady gait

WHAT ARE SOME DIFFERENT TYPES OF TWITCHING, AND HOW DO THEY APPEAR?		
TYPE	WHAT IS IT?	TYPICAL SYMPTOMS
Tics	Rapid, repetitive movements, such as blinking, sniffing, or contracting one side of the face	Tics are more prominent during periods of stress, and can be voluntarily suppressed
Myoclonus	Movements created by involuntary muscle contractions	Rapid, irregular jerks in the arms and legs that occur when falling asleep; these movements may also occur in people with convulsive disorders or nervous system diseases
Chorea	A condition marked by uncontrolled movements throughout the body	Widespread, rapid, and jerky movements in different body regions, skin rash, may occur in children after joint pain and fever; these movements may also occur in people with nervous system diseases or those taking certain medications
Fasciculations	Brief, nonrhythmic contractions of muscles	Small contractions that make the muscle appear to shiver, common in fatigued muscles

Skin Problems

What it feels like: patches of abnormal skin that may itch or blister and appear scaly or crusty.

What can make it worse: scratching, contact with an irritant such as poison ivy or wool.

Your Doctor Visit

What your doctor will ask you about: fever, chills, any previous skin diagnoses, the results of previous skin biopsies, effects of past treatment with antihistamines, steroid pills, or creams.

Your doctor will want to know if you or anyone in your family has had any of these conditions: diabetes, kidney disease, asthma, hay fever, skin diseases such as eczema, psoriasis, or contact dermatitis.

Your doctor will want to know how the problem started, how it has changed over time, how many regions of skin are affected, and if the problem appears to be healing or spreading.

Your doctor will want to know if you're taking any medications.

Your doctor will ask about any recent contact with someone with a similar problem, the nature of your work, and if you ever come into contact with certain dusts, chemicals, or pets.

Your doctor will do a physical examination including the following: temperature, thorough skin examination.

WHAT ARE DIFFERENT TYPES OF SKIN PROBLEMS, AND HOW DO THEY APPEAR?

COMMON SKIN PROBLEMS IN ADULTS

PROBLEM	WHAT IS IT?	TYPICAL SYMPTOMS
Eczema	A rash that can appear in response to allergies, poor circulation, or sunlight	Redness, crust, scales
Wart	Bump on the skin caused by a virus	Occurs often on the hands and feet, most common in children and young adults
Acne	Inflammation of the glands and hair follicles, producing pimples	Blackheads, whiteheads, elevated spots filled with pus; most often found on the face, back, chest, and shoulders
Fungal infection, scalp	Invasion of fungus in the skin of the scalp	Scaling red patches, hair loss, broken hairs
Fungal infection, body	Invasion of fungus in the skin	Itching, scaling, inflamed patches of skin, blisters, may heal in the center but spread, forming a ring
Fungal infection, groin	Invasion of fungus in the skin around the groin	Itchy, red, scaly, spreads to other skin regions
Fungal infection, feet and hands	Invasion of fungus in the skin of the hands and feet	Itchy, blisters on the palms of the hands and soles of the feet, scaling and tears in between toes
Psoriasis	Disease marked by recurrent episodes of itchy, red, and scaly skin	Patches on the scalp or knees or elbows, often itchy, may spread to nails, groin, or entire torso; occurs only in adults
Seborrheic dermatitis	White or yellow scales on the skin, which may flake off; also known as dandruff	Scaly patches on the scalp, eyebrows, back of ears, upper lip, chest, or groin

**WHAT ARE DIFFERENT TYPES OF SKIN PROBLEMS,
AND HOW DO THEY APPEAR? (CONTINUED)**

COMMON SKIN PROBLEMS IN ADULTS

PROBLEM	WHAT IS IT?	TYPICAL SYMPTOMS
Impetigo	Contagious skin disease caused by bacteria	Red spots and blisters that blend together to form a honey-colored crust; occurs in children, most often on the head, neck, and diaper area
Boils	Swollen spots caused by a bacterial infection of a hair follicle	Tender spots normally found in skin regions that contain hair
Hives (See chapter on Allergic Symptoms.)	Raised, red welts on the skin surface	Itchy and pink patches of skin; may occur after eating shellfish or unusual foods, or after taking certain drugs
Scabies	Contagious skin condition caused by mites	Itchy spots and blisters often found in warm body regions, such as between fingers, near the nipples, navel, knees, and groin
Lice	Contagious skin condition caused by wingless insects	Itchy spots, hives (see above), bloody crusts on skin regions with hair
Pityriasis rosea	Rash of unknown cause	Oval, salmon-colored scaly patches of skin on the trunk; occurs mostly in young adults
Yeast infection	Skin inflammation caused by yeast	Red and moist skin spots, itchy, painful. Occurs most often in diabetics and children, and on moist skin regions, such as the groin and base of the nails

**WHAT ARE DIFFERENT TYPES OF SKIN PROBLEMS,
AND HOW DO THEY APPEAR? (CONTINUED)**

*COMMON RASHES SEEN IN CHILDREN (ALSO SEE CHAPTER ON DIAPER
PROBLEMS)*

PROBLEM	WHAT IS IT?	TYPICAL SYMPTOMS
Papovirus	A virus that often causes warts in adults	Red cheeks, rash on torso, slight fever
Chicken pox	Contagious disease marked by skin spots and caused by a herpes virus	Highly itchy blister-like spots, found primarily on the torso, spots crust over several days after they first appear
German measles	Contagious skin disease that is less severe than measles (see below)	Fever, swollen lymph nodes in the neck, followed by sudden rash on face that fades after one day, and followed by a similar rash on the torso, legs, and arms the next day
Measles	Contagious skin disease caused by a virus	Cough and fever for three days followed by a purple-red rash that starts at the head and spreads to the rest of the body

Sleep Problems

What it feels like: having trouble falling asleep, or waking up early in the morning, before you have fully rested.

What can make it worse: drinking alcohol or caffeinated beverages, smoking, stress, being inactive.

The amount of sleep people need varies, but typically falls between 7 and 8 hours each night. People experience two types of sleep—deep sleep and lighter sleep, when they dream. As people age, they tend to spend less time in deep sleep, perhaps explaining why older people often wake up several times each night and are considered "light sleepers."

Some cases of sleep problems occur for simple reasons, such as inactivity or boredom, leading you to take naps and therefore struggle to sleep at night.

Your Doctor Visit

What your doctor will ask you about: daytime napping, loud snoring, needing to urinate in the middle of the night, anxiety, depression, pains in muscles, chest pain, joint pain, results of interventions you have tried to improve your sleep.

Your doctor will want to know if you or anyone in your family has had any of these conditions: lung disease, heart disease.

Your doctor will want to know when you began to have trouble sleeping, and how many hours of interrupted sleep you typically get each night.

Your doctor will want to know if you're taking any of these medications: diuretics ("water pills"), asthma medications, sedatives, tranquilizers, antidepressants.

Your doctor will do a physical examination including the following: height, weight, checking legs and arms for swelling, testing for any painful body regions.

WHAT CAN CAUSE SLEEP PROBLEMS, AND WHAT IS TYPICAL FOR EACH CAUSE?

CAUSE	WHAT IS IT?	TYPICAL SYMPTOMS
Anxiety, depression	A chronically anxious or depressed mood	Feeling anxious or sad for long periods of time, trouble falling asleep (anxiety or depression), or trouble staying asleep (depression)
Alcohol, sedatives	Drinking alcoholic beverages or taking sedatives	Falling asleep with ease, waking up early before getting enough rest
Stimulant use	Drinking caffeinated beverages, smoking cigarettes, taking asthma medications	Trouble sleeping
Pain-causing illnesses	Arthritis, chest pain that occurs at night	Trouble sleeping because of pain (See chapters on Chest Pain and Joint Pain.)
Illnesses that cause night urination	Prostate disease, heart failure	Trouble sleeping because of the need to get up and urinate at night (See chapter on Urine Problems.)
Illnesses that cause trouble breathing	Lung disease, heart failure	Trouble sleeping because of difficulty breathing (See chapter on Breathing Problems.)
Obstructive sleep apnea	Interruptions to sleep caused by trouble breathing due to airway blockages	Frequent waking during sleep, loud snoring, daytime napping, feeling tired; occurs more commonly in overweight people

Small Baby

What it appears like: a baby is relatively small for his or her age.

Most small babies are genetically small, meaning many of their family members were similarly small when younger. See below for other, less frequent causes of small size in babies.

Your Doctor Visit

What your doctor will ask you about: cough, breathing trouble, trouble exercising, bluish or purplish discoloration of the skin, trouble eating, smelly and greasy bowel movements, vomiting, constipation, diarrhea, fever, behavior problems, tiredness, how long the baby has been small, birth weight, birth height, the baby's growth pattern, any recent changes in growth, weight before and after breast-feeding.

Your doctor will want to know if the baby or anyone in the baby's family has had any of these conditions: any chronic disease, past serious illnesses that have since been "cured," exposure to HIV, small stature, cystic fibrosis, kidney disease.

Your doctor may ask about the baby's dietary history and family life, such as whether there have been any recent births, deaths, or hospitalizations.

Your doctor will want to know if the baby is taking any medications.

Your doctor will do a physical examination of the baby, including the following: weight, height, head size, temperature, pulse, blood pressure, looking inside the throat, listening to the chest and heart with a stethoscope, pushing on the abdomen, checking arms and legs for muscle strength, thorough skin examination, testing reflexes, checking lymph nodes to see if they are enlarged.

WHAT CAN CAUSE SMALL SIZE IN BABIES, AND WHAT IS TYPICAL FOR EACH CAUSE?		
CAUSE	WHAT IS IT?	TYPICAL SYMPTOMS
Inadequate feeding	Lack of nutrients needed to support normal growth	Smaller increase in weight than height, weight loss, protuberant abdomen, caregivers may fear "over-feeding the child"; if the child lives in warm climates, he or she may not be getting enough fluids with meals
Cystic fibrosis	A genetic disease in which the body undergoes changes causing diarrhea, recurrent lung infections, and other problems	Frequent lung infections, smelly and greasy stools, family history of fibrocystic disease, smaller increase in weight than height, weight loss, protuberant abdomen
Enzyme deficiency diseases	Conditions in which the baby lacks a needed protein	Diarrhea, greasy bowel movements, occasional vomiting after consuming milk or other foods, smaller increase in weight than height, weight loss, protuberant abdomen
Hypothyroidism	Underactive thyroid gland	Prolonged yellowing of skin after birth, constipation, mottled skin as newborn
Growth hormone deficiency	Deficiency of a hormone needed for normal growth	Normal birth weight but slow subsequent growth, delayed growth of teeth
Chronic disease	Chronic diseases or infections, such as lung disease, kidney disease, heart disease, HIV infection, intestinal parasites	History of chronic disease, smaller increase in weight than height, weight loss, fever, protuberant abdomen; baby may exhibit problems with the heart, lungs, or abdomen
"Growth lags"	Delays in growth after illness or other bodily stresses	Normal

Swelling

What it feels like: growth or distention in a region of the body, sometimes painful.

What can make it worse: menstruation, certain positions, injury, drugs, certain foods or dust, time of day, pregnancy.

If your swelling can be described as a **"lump,"** and is located in your neck, under your jaw, around your ears, above your collarbone, under your arms, behind your knees and elbows, or in your groin, the lump is likely a **swollen lymph node**.

Swollen lymph nodes can occur **because of injuries or diseases** such as those affecting the mouth, teeth, or lungs.

Your Doctor Visit

What your doctor will ask you about: weight change, shortness of breath, yellowing of skin, itching, tenderness, redness, or aching in swollen area, chronic loose stools, abdominal pain, chills, pain, fever, rashes, results of a recent EKG or chest X-ray, outcomes of tests of kidney and liver function, discharge or change in appearance (lump).

Your doctor will want to know if you or anyone in your family has had any of these conditions: heart disease, kidney disease, varicose veins, anemia, bowel disease, liver disease, allergies, past injury or surgery in the swollen area, tuberculosis, mononucleosis, sore throat, recurrent infections, sexually transmitted disease.

Your doctor will want to know about your diet, and exactly where you are experiencing swelling.

If you have swollen lymph nodes, your doctor will ask if you have recently received any vaccinations, or been exposed to measles, mumps, chicken pox, or sexually transmitted diseases.

Your doctor will want to know if you're taking any of these medications: diuretics, digitalis, steroids, birth control pills, nifedipine (Procardia), diphenylhydantoin (Dilantin).

Your doctor will do a physical examination including the following: blood pressure, pulse, weight, temperature, thorough neck exam, listening to your chest and heart with a stethoscope, pushing on your abdomen, looking at your legs and arms.

If you have a lump, your doctor will check the lump for size, consistency, and tenderness, and examine your lymph nodes.

WHAT CAN CAUSE SWELLING, AND WHAT IS TYPICAL FOR EACH CAUSE?		
CAUSE	**WHAT IS IT?**	**TYPICAL SYMPTOMS**
Cyclic swelling in women	Bloating and body changes that follow the menstrual cycle	Bloating, weight gain, mild swelling
Medication use	Swelling or weight gain caused by medications	Swelling, weight gain
Infection	Invasion by a pathogen	Swelling around site of infection, warmth, redness, tenderness in skin
Hypo-albuminemia	Decrease in a particular protein in the blood	Weight loss, poor diet, chronic diarrhea, enlarged abdomen
Anemia	Deficiency of needed substances in the blood	Pale skin, shortness of breath
Angioedema (See chapter on Allergic Symptoms.)	Allergic disease in which you develop welts on the skin	Sudden swelling, severe shortness of breath, may occur after injury, infection, or exposure to particular foods or dusts
Ascites	An abnormal collection of fluid in the abdomen	Occurs in people with a history of liver disease, cancer, heart disease, or kidney problems

WHAT CAN CAUSE SWELLING, AND WHAT IS TYPICAL FOR EACH CAUSE? (CONTINUED)		
CAUSE	WHAT IS IT?	TYPICAL SYMPTOMS
Organ failure	Failure of the heart, kidneys, or liver to function properly	Trouble breathing, history of heart, kidney, or liver disease
Toxemia of pregnancy	A dangerous condition during pregnancy that involves high blood pressure	High blood pressure, occurs only in pregnancy
Lymphatic blockage	A block in the vessels that drain fluid from tissues and transport immune cells around the body	Swelling in extremities, may occur after a tumor, surgery, radiation treatment, or infection with a parasite
Venous disease	Problems in the blood vessels, such as inflammation and blockages	Chronic aching, night cramps, itching, painful swelling, brown-purple discoloration of skin

WHAT CAN CAUSE LUMPS OR SWOLLEN LYMPH NODES, AND WHAT IS TYPICAL FOR EACH CAUSE?		
CAUSE	WHAT IS IT?	TYPICAL SYMPTOMS
Infection	Invasion by a virus such as German measles, mumps, mononucleosis, chicken pox	Fever, skin rash, area is tender and warm (See chapter on Skin Problems.)
Malignancy (cancer)	Abnormal, unchecked cell growth	Weight loss, fever, infections, bleeding

Lumps and swelling in lymph nodes are often harmless and pose no danger. Lymph nodes often swell as a result of problems in nearby regions of the body. For instance, swollen nodes in the neck are often a response to dental cavities or other oral problems, while lymph nodes in the thigh or groin can swell in response to infections in the foot, leg, or groin.

Testicle Problems

What it feels like: pain or swelling in the testicles.

What can make it better: lying flat.

Your Doctor Visit

What your doctor will ask you about: undescended or overly mobile testicles, testicular pain or swelling, masses, fever, chills, nausea, pain with or trouble urinating, blood in urine, abnormal skin patches on the scrotum, swollen lymph nodes.

Your doctor will want to know if you or anyone in your family has had any of these conditions: hernia (see below), mumps, kidney stones.

Your doctor will want to know the exact nature of your testicle problems, when they started, and whether you regularly check your testicles for masses.

Your doctor will want to know if you're taking any medications.

Your doctor will do a physical examination including the following: temperature, digital rectal exam, checking for the presence of a hernia in the groin, checking testicles for the presence of a mass.

WHAT CAN CAUSE TESTICLE PROBLEMS, AND WHAT IS TYPICAL FOR EACH CAUSE?

PAIN

CAUSE	WHAT IS IT?	TYPICAL SYMPTOMS
Infection	Invasion of the testicles by bacteria or a virus	Trouble urinating, tenderness, swelling, fever, may begin in the course of hours, may occur following a case of the mumps
Torsion of the testicle	Twisting of the testicle	Sudden onset of severe pain, nausea, tenderness, swelling; occurs most commonly in men between the ages of 5 and 20
Pain referred to the scrotum	Pain in other parts of the body that radiates to the scrotum, or sac that carries the testicles	Pain in the sides of the body, often blood in the urine

TESTICULAR MASS

CAUSE	WHAT IS IT?	TYPICAL SYMPTOMS
Hydrocele	Accumulation of fluid in the scrotum	Noticeable and painless mass, may enlarge when crying
Spermatocele	Swelling in the scrotum	Noticeable and painless mass that is separate from testicle
Varicocele	Swelling of the veins, producing a mass in the scrotum	Noticeable and painless mass, any discomfort disappears when lying down, mass may feel like a "bag of worms"
Tumor	Unchecked, abnormal growth of cells	Noticeable and painless mass connected to the testicle

WHAT CAN CAUSE TESTICLE PROBLEMS, AND WHAT IS TYPICAL FOR EACH CAUSE? (CONTINUED)

TESTICULAR MASS

CAUSE	WHAT IS IT?	TYPICAL SYMPTOMS
Hernia	Condition in which a portion of the intestine pokes through an opening in the abdominal muscles	Noticeable and painless mass, may "fall back" into the abdomen

OTHER

CAUSE	WHAT IS IT?	TYPICAL SYMPTOMS
Absent or undescended testicles	Lack of testicles, testicles may fail to drop down	Occurs in children, testicles may appear pulled into the groin, testicles often descend by 1 year of age

Urine Problems

What it feels like: varies from changes in urine color, to pain with urination, to the inability to control when you urinate.

If your concern is related to changes in the color of your urine, be aware that eating beets can turn urine red, and urine can become dark yellow as a result of fever or dehydration. However, other conditions can cause the same symptoms.

Your Doctor Visit

What your doctor will ask you about: lower back or abdominal pain, vaginal discharge, passing stones or "gravel," fever or chills, pain on urination or frequent urination, urgent need to urinate, dark or bloody urine, decreased force of urine stream, urination at night, uncontrolled urination, recent trauma to the anal region or abdomen, bruising or bleeding, pale stools, jaundice (skin taking on a yellowish appearance).

Your doctor will want to know if you or anyone in your family has had any of these conditions: kidney stones, kidney disease, recurrent urinary tract infections, bladder or prostate disease, diabetes, neurologic disease, high blood pressure, liver disease, blood disease, sickle-cell disease, anemia.

Your doctor will want to know if you're taking any medications, including: antibiotics, warfarin (Coumadin), urinary painkillers such as pyridium.

Your doctor will do a physical examination including the following: temperature, blood pressure, pushing on your abdomen, digital rectal exam, checking limbs for swelling and reflexes, testing reflexes and movement, thorough skin exam.

WHAT CAN CAUSE URINE PROBLEMS, AND WHAT IS TYPICAL FOR EACH CAUSE?		
CAUSE	**WHAT IS IT?**	**TYPICAL SYMPTOMS**
Hematuria	Blood in urine, resulting from other conditions	Dark urine, sometimes no other symptoms, sometimes painful urination, abdominal or flank pain, changes in urinary habits

PAINFUL URINATION

CAUSE	WHAT IS IT?	TYPICAL SYMPTOMS
Cystitis	Bladder infection or inflammation	Fever, an urgent need to urinate, frequent urination, chills, sometimes blood in urine
Pyelonephritis	Kidney infection	Frequent urination, flank pain, fever and chills
Urethritis (men)	Inflammation in the ureter resulting from infection, such as by the bacteria that cause gonorrhea	Watery discharge from penis
Kidney stones	The presence of a stone made up of mineral salts in the kidney	History of passing blood or "gravel" in urine, severe pain radiating to groin or testicle
Prostatitis	Prostate infection or inflammation	Changes in urination, lower abdominal pain

TROUBLE URINATING

CAUSE	WHAT IS IT?	TYPICAL SYMPTOMS
Acute urinary retention	Inability to urinate	Lower abdominal discomfort, history of prostate trouble or kidney stones, sometimes occurs after taking anticholinergic medications such as Benadryl

WHAT CAN CAUSE URINE PROBLEMS,
AND WHAT IS TYPICAL FOR EACH CAUSE? (CONTINUED)

TROUBLE URINATING

Cause	What Is It?	Typical Symptoms
Urethral obstruction	A blockage in the tube that drains urine from the bladder, usually the result of prostate problems	Difficulty initiating urinating, frequent urinating, decreased force of urine stream, most common in older men

UNCONTROLLED URINATION

Cause	What Is It?	Typical Symptoms
Stress incontinence	Leaking urine with laughing, coughing, or straining	Most common in women after multiple pregnancies
Incontinence due to neurological problem	Leaking urine as a result of problems in the nervous system	Low back pain, history of diabetes, stroke, or dementia; lower extremities may be weak, painful, or numb

FREQUENT URINATION AT NIGHT

Cause	What Is It?	Typical Symptoms
Diuretic ("water pills") use	Too much fluid in the body, a result of taking diuretics such as Lasix or hydrochlorothiazide, both used to control high blood pressure, or the result of drinking coffee or alcohol before bed	The need to urinate wakens you
Fluid retention	Too much fluid in the body, a result of conditions such as congestive heart failure	Shortness of breath, swelling in the legs
Diabetes	High levels of sugar in the blood	Weight loss, frequent urination during the day as well as at night

Vaginal Bleeding Problems

What it feels like: varies from lack of or painful monthly periods to excessive or abnormal bleeding while menstruating.

Your Doctor Visit

What your doctor will ask you about: emotional stress, anxiety, depression, hot flashes, changes in weight, heat intolerance, changes in the distribution or texture of hair, breast enlargement, nausea, vomiting, abdominal pain, fever, chills, bruising, passing "tissue" in menstrual blood, results of previous thyroid tests, Pap tests, and pelvic exams.

Your doctor will want to know if you or anyone in your family has had any of these conditions: pelvic inflammatory disease, diabetes, thyroid disease, drug addiction, emotional disease, pregnancies, miscarriages, abortions, bleeding problems.

Your doctor will ask you how many menstrual pads you use each day you are bleeding, the date of your last menstrual period, and whether your bleeding occurs around the time you should get your period.

Your doctor will want to know if there is a chance you are pregnant.

Your doctor will want to know the age at which you began to grow body hair and breasts, when you menstruated for the first time, and the age of your mother and any sisters when they began and stopped menstruating.

Your doctor will want to know if you're taking any of these medications: birth control pills, intrauterine device, warfarin (Coumadin), thyroid pills, steroids.

Your doctor will do a physical examination including the following: blood pressure, pulse, temperature, pelvic exam, Pap test, thorough skin exam.

What are different types of vaginal bleeding problems, and what is typical for each?		
Problem	**What Is It?**	**Typical Causes**
Amenorrhea	Lack of menstrual periods	Delayed puberty, diabetes, anorexia nervosa, thyroid disease, inherited disorder, pregnancy, a wide variety of other diseases
Dysmenorrhea (See chapter on Menstrual Cramps.)	Painful menstrual periods	A common problem in otherwise healthy women; for some women, dysmenorrhea is a symptom of endometriosis—the growth of tissue from the uterus in places other than the uterus—or pelvic inflammatory disease, caused by sexually transmitted diseases (See chapters on Sexually Transmitted Diseases (STDs) and Sexual Problems and Inability to Conceive.)
Abnormal bleeding	Too much or irregular bleeding	A common problem for healthy women who are menstruating for the first or last times; for some women, abnormal bleeding is a sign of a problem in early pregnancy, tumors in the cervix or uterus, or a wide variety of other disorders

Vaginal Discharge

What it feels like: a white, clear, or colored discharge from the vagina, sometimes accompanied by itching or a foul odor.

What can make it worse: having sex with a person with a sexually transmitted disease, pregnancy, having a foreign object in the vagina.

Clear discharge is often normal in children.

Your Doctor Visit

What your doctor will ask you about: fever or chills, abdominal pain, itching around the vagina or anus, redness or tenderness in the vagina, smelly discharge, pain or difficulty with urination, joint pain, skin rash, the date of your last pelvic exam and Pap smear, douching, recent intercourse with a person with a sexually transmitted disease, the presence of a foreign body in your vagina.

Your doctor will want to know if you or anyone in your family has had any of these conditions: gonorrhea, syphilis, vaginitis, diabetes.

Your doctor will want to know about the color of your discharge, how much discharge you are experiencing, and its relationship to your menstrual cycle.

Your doctor will want to know if you're taking any of these medications: oral contraceptives, antibiotics.

Your doctor will do a physical examination including the following: pushing on your abdomen, pelvic exam, Pap test.

WHAT CAN CAUSE VAGINAL DISCHARGE, AND WHAT IS TYPICAL FOR EACH CAUSE?		
CAUSE	**WHAT IS IT?**	**TYPICAL SYMPTOMS**
Candidiasis	Yeast infection	Itching, white discharge, more common in diabetics, pregnant women, and women using oral contraceptives or antibiotics
Gonorrhea (See chapter on Sexually Transmitted Diseases.)	Sexually transmitted disease caused by the bacterium *Neisseria gonorrhoeae*	Abdominal pain, fever, chills, joint pain, history of sex with an infected person
Mixed bacteria	Vaginal bacterial infection	Often history of excessive douching, foul odor, some itching, sometimes a foreign body is present in the vagina
Chlamydia	Vaginal infection caused by *Chlamydia trachomatis*, a bacterium	Clear, watery discharge, spotting of blood after intercourse
Trichomoniasis	Sexually transmitted disease caused by a parasite	Severe itching, heavy discharge, discharge is frothy, gray, green, or yellow
Endometrial cancer	Unchecked, abnormal growth of cells in tissue from the uterus	Light discharge, sometimes discharge contains blood, abdominal tenderness

Weakness

What it feels like: tiredness, weakness, or giddiness, sometimes more pronounced while standing, which can be the result of an underlying condition or disease, such as anemia (see below) or an infection.

What can make it worse: exertion, certain medications, and stress related to family, job, or school problems.

In adults, a very common cause of weakness or tiredness is depression, manifested as trouble waking up, the feeling that small tasks are large obstacles, emotional instability, and difficulty sleeping or concentrating. If you think you may have depression, see the chapter on Depression, Suicidal Thoughts, or Anxiety for more details. Other associated symptoms mentioned here — such as swollen lymph nodes — may prompt your doctor to look into other causes such as infection or cancer. See the chapter on Swelling for more information.

Your Doctor Visit

What your doctor will ask you about: diet, weight loss, weakness or dizziness when standing, bruising, vomiting blood, black stools, diarrhea, excessive menstrual bleeding, tiredness on arising in the morning, trouble concentrating, loss of appetite, loss of interest in sex, fever or chills, sore throat, difficulty breathing, headache, chest or abdominal pain, muscle weakness, excessive sleeping. He or she will also ask whether you have ever been told you are anemic, and whether you have ever had a bone marrow biopsy (a procedure in which a long needle is inserted into a bone near your hip), and if so, what the results were.

Your doctor will want to know if you or anyone in your family has had any emotional disorders or chronic diseases.

Your doctor will want to know if you're taking any medications, including: methyldopa (Aldomet), reserpine, beta-blockers, seda-

tives, tranquilizers, antidepressants, antihistamines, aspirin, ibuprofen or other nonsteroidal anti-inflammatory drugs, steroids, iron,
vitamin B12, folate.

**Your doctor will do a physical examination including the follow-
ing:** blood pressure, pulse, temperature, weight, checking your throat
for redness, listening to your heart and chest with a stethoscope, pushing on your abdomen, checking your lymph nodes to see if they are
enlarged, testing your stool for blood, eye exam, thorough skin exam.

WHAT CAN CAUSE WEAKNESS, AND WHAT IS TYPICAL FOR EACH CAUSE?		
CAUSE	**WHAT LEADS TO IT?**	**TYPICAL SYMPTOMS**
Extreme blood loss	Sudden injury, or internal bleeding due to a tumor or other condition	Fatigue, weakness, bleeding, tar-like stools, pallor
Iron deficiency	Menstruation or poor diet	Fatigue, weakness
Folate (a B vitamin) deficiency	Alcoholism or poor diet	Fatigue, weakness
Vitamin B12 deficiency	Poor absorption of vitamin B12, which is sometimes hereditary	Fatigue, diarrhea, reduced sensation in toes
Failure of the bone marrow (the place your body makes most blood cells)	Chronic disease including some kinds of cancers, exposure to chemicals such as benzene or arsenic, exposure to radiation, chemotherapy, gold shots (given for arthritis)	Fatigue, weakness
Increased destruction of blood cells	Sickle-cell anemia, malaria, recent transfusion, family history of anemia	Fatigue, weakness, jaundice (skin taking on a yellowish appearance)

Yellow Skin

What it feels like: skin taking on a yellowish appearance, also called jaundice.

What can make it worse: taking certain medications, intravenous drugs, drinking alcohol, exposure to chemical solvents, receiving blood products.

Jaundice occurs when you accumulate too much of a substance called bilirubin, which results from the breakdown of red blood cells, in the blood. Almost every newborn has at least a mild case of jaundice, which typically causes no problems.

Your Doctor Visit

What your doctor will ask you about: headache, loss of appetite, nausea, vomiting, fever, shaking chills, abdominal pain, change in weight, abdominal swelling, black or tarry stools, blood in stools, light-colored stools, dark urine, change in thinking patterns, joint pain, itchiness, results of tests related to the problem, including a liver biopsy.

Your doctor will want to know if you or anyone in your family has had any of these conditions: jaundice, alcoholism, gallstones, liver disease, past gastrointestinal bleeding, drug addiction, mononucleosis, blood disease, cancer.

Your doctor will want to know when you first noticed your symptoms, and if you have had close contact with another person with jaundice, if you work with chemical solvents, or if you have traveled within the past six months.

Your doctor will want to know if you're taking any medications, including: isoniazid (for tuberculosis), phenothiazine antipsychotics such as Haldol, oral contraceptives, recent anesthetics, cholesterol-lowering drugs, sulfa antibiotics such as sulfamethoxa-zole, the antibiotic nitrofurantoin, the heart drug quinidine.

Your doctor will do a physical examination including the following: blood pressure, pulse, temperature, pushing on the abdomen, checking stool for the presence of blood, checking size of testicles and breasts (male), thorough skin examination. Your doctor may also ask you questions to check your mental status, such as if you know where you are and recent events.

WHAT CAN CAUSE YELLOW SKIN, AND WHAT IS TYPICAL FOR EACH CAUSE?		
CAUSE	**WHAT IS IT?**	**TYPICAL SYMPTOMS**
Viral hepatitis	Infection of the liver caused by a virus such as hepatitis A, B, or C; hepatitis B and C are more common in intravenous drug abusers and people who were in contact with blood products, other jaundiced people, or contaminated water; hepatitis A can be contracted from food and is less severe	Jaundice begins over days and weeks, upper abdominal pain, nausea, vomiting, joint pain, fever, headache, dark urine, light stools
Toxic hepatitis	Inflammation of the liver caused by alcohol, drugs, or chemical solvents	Jaundice begins over days and weeks, dark urine, light stools, upper abdominal pain
Obstruction of biliary flow	Blockage in the flow of digestive fluid that contains bilirubin from the liver, causing a buildup of bilirubin in the blood	Itching, light stools, dark urine, history of gallstones
Gilbert's syndrome	Inherited disorder that affects the processing of bilirubin	Jaundice occurs in periods of exercise, fasting, stress, or infection
Dubin-Johnson syndrome	Inherited disorder that affects the transport of bilirubin	Mild jaundice throughout entire life, begins after puberty

WHAT CAN CAUSE YELLOW SKIN, AND WHAT IS TYPICAL FOR EACH CAUSE? (CONTINUED)		
CAUSE	WHAT IS IT?	TYPICAL SYMPTOMS
Chronic liver disease	Long-term liver disease, causing scarring of the liver, also known as cirrhosis, often caused by a long history of alcoholism	Chronic jaundice, history of any of the listed causes of jaundice, red palms
Liver failure	Inability of the liver to function properly	History of infection or gastrointestinal bleeding with liver disease, disorientation, stupor, coma

IN INFANTS, THE TIME WHEN JAUNDICE APPEARS CAN HELP DETERMINE THE CAUSE.

YELLOW SKIN IN INFANTS

TIME OF APPEARANCE	CAUSES
24 hours after birth	Breakdown of blood cells or any of the causes listed above
Between 2 and 4 days after birth	Normal, will disappear eventually; if it persists beyond a week, it may be due to a more serious liver or gland problem
Fifth or later day after birth	Severe infection

Glossary

Included below are *simple* definitions of key words used in the text.

ABRASION—superficial scraping of skin.

ABSCESS—a localized collection of pus.

ACUTE—sudden; having a short course.

ADRENAL—a gland near the kidney that is important in the body's reaction to stress.

AIDS—acquired immunodeficiency syndrome. A disease resulting from infection with the human immunodeficiency virus (HIV).

AMBLYOPIA—a condition in which a "lazy" eye does not fix accurately on objects; may eventually cause squint (cross-eyes, walleyes) and blindness of the "lazy" eye.

ANALGESIA—absence (or decrease) of pain sensation.

ANEMIA—deficiency of blood quantity or quality.

ANGINA—a pattern of chest pain usually due to disease of the heart's arteries.

ANGIOPLASTY—use of a catheter to stretch a narrow region of an artery.

ANKYLOSING SPONDYLITIS—a disease of young men causing persistent back pain eventually resulting in fixation of the spine.

ANOREXIA—loss of appetite.

ANOREXIA NERVOSA—a disease in which the patient refuses to maintain a normal weight and may die of starvation.

ANTIARRHYTHMICS—medications used to regulate the abnormal beating of the heart.

ANTIBIOTICS—medications used to help the body fight bacterial or fungal infections.

ANTIBODY—a blood protein (globulin) useful in helping the body fight infections.

ANTICHOLINERGICS—medications that block nerves that help activate digestive processes.

ANTICONVULSANTS—medications used to control convulsive (seizure) disorders.

ANTISPASMODICS—see *Anticholinergics*, above.

APHASIA—loss of the ability to speak or write because of brain damage.

ARRHYTHMIA—abnormal beat of the heart.

ARTERIOGRAM—an x-ray study of dye injected into vessels carrying blood away from the heart.

ARTHRALGIA—joint aches causing no joint tenderness or destruction.

ASCITES—an abnormal collection of fluid in the abdomen (peritoneal cavity).

ASYMPTOMATIC—referring to a disease causing no patient complaints.

ATAXIA—unsteadiness; incoordination.

ATHEROSCLEROSIS—"hardening" of the arteries.

ATRIAL—pertaining to the two upper chambers of the heart that receive blood from the body and lungs.

AUTONOMIC—the involuntary part of the nervous system that controls bodily functions such as digestion or blood pressure.

AXILLA—armpit.

BARIUM ENEMA—x-ray of the large bowel.

BETA-BLOCKING AGENT—medications, such as propranolol, that block the sympathetic nervous system beta receptors causing, for example, a reduced heart rate.

BILIARY—the drainage system of the liver (bile ducts, gallbladder).

BIOPSY—surgical removal of tissue for examination.

BIRTH TRAUMA—injury to the infant during birth.

BRONCHIECTASIS—chronic dilatations in the air passage ways to the lungs.

BRONCHODILATORS—medications that can dilate the air passages in the lung.

BURSITIS—inflammation of the lubricating sac near a joint.

CALCIUM CHANNEL AGENTS—medications, such as verapamil and nifedipine, that may reduce vascular spasm and often have associated antiarrhythmic and antihypertensive effects.

CARDIOVASCULAR—pertaining to the heart and blood vessels.

CT (CAT) SCAN—a radiologic method for examining cross sections of the body.

CATHETER—a tube for withdrawing fluids from, or putting fluids into, the body.

CEREBROVASCULAR—pertaining to the blood vessels directly supplying the brain.

CHOLESTEROL and TRIGLYCERIDES—fatlike substances in the blood.

CHRONIC—not acute, of long duration.

CIRRHOSIS—scarring of the liver.

CLAUDICATION—calf pain caused by inadequate blood supply (*see* JOINT PAIN, page 138).

COLIC—*see* ABDOMINAL PAIN (child), page 6.

COLITIS—inflammatory disease of the large bowel.

COMA—unconsciousness.

COLONOSCOPY—visualization of the large bowel by passing a flexible tube through the anus.

CONGESTIVE HEART FAILURE—failure of heart function causing the body to retain fluid; fluid retention often causes edema of the legs, shortness of breath, and abnormal sounds in the lungs (rales).

CONJUNCTIVITIS—inflammation of the membrane that lines the eyelids and overlies the "whites" of the eyes.

CONTACT DERMATITIS—skin inflammation caused by touching certain substances.

CONNECTIVE TISSUE DISEASE—disease of the tissue that supports most structures of the body (e.g., connective tissue is found in joints, blood vessels, tendons, skin, and muscles).

COSTOVERTEBRAL ANGLE—see *Flank*.

CYANOSIS—blue-colored skin due to insufficient oxygen in the blood.

CYST—a sac containing fluid.

CYSTIC FIBROSIS—a hereditary chronic disease often causing greasy foul—smelling diarrhea, recurrent lung infections, and death.

DEFECATION—the process of having a bowel movement.

DELIRIUM—a confused state due to underlying disease.

DELIRIUM TREMENS—delirium due to cessation of chronic alcohol ingestion.

DEMENTIA—usually irreversible mental deterioration.

DENTITION—referring to the teeth.

DERMATITIS—inflammation of the skin.

DESENSITIZATION—causing a person to no longer react to a substance.

DIAGNOSIS—a description of an illness usually based on a combination of symptoms and findings.

DIAPHORESIS—profuse sweating.

DIGITALIS—a drug useful for strengthening the heart.

DIPLOPIA—double vision.

DISTAL—farthest from the body.

DISTENTION—being swollen or stretched.

DIURETICS—"water" pills; medications that cause increased urine secretion.

DIVERTICULA—small blind pouches most often found extending from the wall of the large bowel or esophagus.

DYSGENESIS—defective development.

DYSFUNCTION—abnormal function.

DYSMENORRHEA—painful menstrual periods.

DYSPAREUNIA—painful sexual intercourse in women.

DYSPHAGIA—difficulty swallowing.

DYSPNEA—the sensation of being short of breath.

DYSURIA—painful urination.

ECCHYMOSES—bruises.

ECHO—See *Sonogram*.

ECZEMA—*see* SKIN PROBLEMS, page 186.

EDEMA—an abnormal increase in tissue fluid; edema is clinically apparent in the lungs or under the skin.

EMBOLUS—a blood clot that moves through the blood vessels.

EMPHYSEMA—a form of chronic lung disease.

ENCEPHALITIS—inflammation or infection of the brain.

ENDOCARDITIS—inflammation or infection of the heart.

ENDOMETRIOSIS—tissue from the uterus that collects in abnormal places.

ENDOSCOPY—visualization of the upper or lower gastrointestinal tract by using a flexible tube.

ENURESIS—bed-wetting.

ENTERITIS—inflammation of the small bowel.

EPIGLOTTITIS—inflammation of a structure in the throat (the epiglottis) that can block the air passages.

EPIGASTRIUM—the upper middle portion of the abdomen.

EPISTAXIS—nosebleed.

ERUCTATION—a burp.

ERYTHEMA—redness.

EXCORIATION—scratching away of superficial skin.

EXOPHTHALMOS—bulging of the eyeballs.

EXPECTORATION—coughing up a substance.

EXUDATE—a fluid that often forms on injured surfaces and turns into a yellow crust when dry.

FECAL—pertaining to bowel movements.

FEMORAL—pertaining to structures on or near the thigh bone.

FIBRILLATION—fine spontaneous contraction of muscles.

FIBROCYSTIC—see *Cystic fibrosis*.

FIBROID (LEIOMYOMA)—a nonmalignant muscular growth of the uterus.

FIBROSIS—scarring.

FISTULA—an abnormal passage; usually from the skin to an internal structure.

FLANK—the lateral back sides of the abdomen.

FLATULENCE—the passage of gas.

FOLATE—a vitamin.

GASTRIC—pertaining to the stomach.

GASTROENTERITIS—acute upset of bowel function.

GASTROINTESTINAL—pertaining to the stomach and bowels.

GASTROSCOPY—visualization of the stomach using a long tube.

GIDDY—light-headed.

GLAUCOMA—abnormal high pressure in the eyeball.

GLOBULIN—a type of protein in the body.

GONOCOCCAL—pertaining to the bacteria causing gonorrhea.

GOUT—a disease causing acute painful joints; usually in men.

GROSS—coarse or large.

GYNECOMASTIA—enlarged breasts.

HEAT STROKE—*see* HEAT STROKE, page 117.

HEMATEMESIS—vomiting blood.

HEMATURIA—blood in urine.

HEMOPHILIA—a hereditary disease caused by a reduced ability of blood to form clots.

HEMOPTYSIS—coughing blood.

HEPATITIS—inflammation of the liver.

HEPATOMEGALY—large liver.

HEPATOSPLENOMEGALY—large liver and spleen.

HESITANCY—inability to begin urinating.

HIATUS HERNIA—an opening allowing the stomach to slide into the chest.

HIRSUTISM—abnormal hairiness.

HIV—see *AIDS*.

HOT FLASHES—the sensation of fever associated with the menopause.

HYDROCEPHALUS—abnormal collection of fluid in the skull causing brain damage.

HYPERTENSION—abnormal elevation of blood pressure.

HYPERVENTILATION—prolonged rapid and deep breathing.

HYPOGLYCEMIA—low blood sugar.

HYPOPLASTIC—incompletely developed.

HYPOREFLEXIA—weak reflexes.

HYPOTENSION—abnormally low blood pressure.

INCONTINENCE—inability to control bladder or bowel.

INFARCTION—death of tissue due to poor blood supply.

INFLAMMATION—the reaction of body tissues to injury characterized by swelling, warmth, tenderness, and, when visible, redness.

INGUINAL—pertaining to the groin.

ISCHEMIA—a local or temporary lack of blood to tissue.

JAUNDICE—abnormal yellow skin (see YELLOW SKIN, page 208).

KETOACIDOSIS—a state in which a person lacks sufficient substances in the blood (insulin). Often results in coma, dehydration, and abnormal acidification of the body fluids. Usually a problem of persons suffering from insulin-dependent diabetes.

LACERATION—a cut.

LACTATION—nursing; secretion of milk.

LESION—an abnormality (usually of the skin).

LETHARGY—strictly defined as drowsiness; often means "feeling tired out" (lassitude) in common usage.

LEUKOCYTE—white blood cell in body that helps fight infections.

LUMBAR PUNCTURE—placing a needle into the lower spine to withdraw fluid that surrounds the spinal cord.

LUPUS ERYTHEMATOSUS—a connective tissue disease.

LYMPH NODES—absorbent glandlike structures that collect drainage of a clear fluid from the body.

LYMPHADENOPATHY—enlargement of lymph nodes.

MALAISE—fatigue; generalized body discomfort.

MALIGNANCY—a disease tending to go from bad to worse; usually a cancer.

MELENA—black, tarry bowel movements.

MÉNIÈRE'S DISEASE—*see* DIZZINESS, page 72.

MENINGITIS—infection or inflammation of the covering of the brain.

MENORRHAGIA—heavy menstrual bleeding.

MENSES—menstrual periods.

MRI—Magnetic resonance imaging. A radiologic technique used to study the body.

MYALGIA—muscle aches.

MYELOGRAM—an x-ray study of dye injected around the spinal cord.

MYOCARDIAL INFARCTION—death of heart muscle due to an inadequate blood supply.

MYOGRAM—electrical measurement of muscle activity.

NASOGASTRIC INTUBATION—the passage of a tube from the nose to the stomach.

NECROSIS—death.

NEURODERMATITIS—nervous scratching.

NEUROLOGIC—pertaining to the nervous system.

NEUROPATHY—disease of nerves.

NOCTURIA—having to urinate at night.

NODE—a lymph gland.

OBSTIPATION—severe constipation.

OBSTRUCTIVE PULMONARY DISEASE—a common form of chronic lung disease (emphysema).

ORCHITIS—inflammation of testicles.

ORTHOPNEA—inability to breathe when lying down; relieved by sitting up.

ORTHOSTATIC—caused by standing up.

OSTEOARTHRITIS—the common arthritis of old age (degenerative arthritis).

OTITIS MEDIA—infection of the middle ear.

PALPITATION—sensation of heart beat.

PANCREATITIS—inflammation of the pancreas.

PARESTHESIA—an abnormal sensation (tingling, prickling, etc.).

PELVIC INFLAMMATORY DISEASE—usually gonorrhea.

PEPTIC ULCER—ulcer of the stomach, duodenum, or lower esophagus.

PERICARDIUM—the sac surrounding the heart.

PERINEAL—the area between the thighs.

PERIORAL—around the mouth.

PERIRECTAL—around the rectum.

PERITONEUM—the space between the bowels and the abdominal wall.

PETECHIAE—spot-sized bleeding into the skin.

PHARYNGITIS—inflammation of the posterior throat.

PHENOTHIAZINES—medications that tend to sedate and to control psychotic thoughts.

PHLEBITIS—inflammation of veins; blood clot is usually present.

PHOTOPHOBIA—abnormal intolerance of light.

PLEURISY—inflammation of the covering of the lungs; usually painful.

PNEUMOTHORAX—an abnormal collection of air between the lungs and the chest wall.

POLYDIPSIA—excessive thirst (amount).

POLYP—a growth that protrudes into a cavity (e.g., nasal polyp, polyp of large bowel).

POLYPHAGIA—excessive appetite.

POLYURIA—excessive urination (amount).

POPLITEAL—the space behind the knee.

POSTPRANDIAL—after meals.

PRECORDIAL—region overlying the heart.

PRIMARY—first in order; principal.

PROCTOSCOPE—visualization of the lower bowel by passing a tube through the anus.

PRODROME—a symptom indicating the beginning of a disease.

PROLAPSE—falling out of position.

PRURITUS—itching.

PSORIASIS—*see* SKIN PROBLEMS, page 186.

PULMONARY—pertaining to lungs.

PULSATILE—rhythmic movement.

PURULENT—containing pus.

PUSTULE—a small skin elevation filled with pus.

PYELOGRAM—an x-ray study of the kidneys after injecting dye into the blood.

RECTUM—the last portion of the large bowel.

RENAL—pertaining to kidneys.

RHEUMATIC FEVER—a disease, usually of children, with fever, joint pains, and possible heart damage.

RHEUMATOID ARTHRITIS—a deforming chronic disease of joints.

RHINITIS—inflammation of the inside of the nose.

SCAPULA—shoulder blade.

SCLERAL ICTERUS—yellowing of the "whites" of the eyes.

SECONDARY—second or inferior in order.

SECONDARY SEXUAL CHARACTERISTICS—sexual characteristics occurring at puberty that differentiate male from female (voice changes, muscle changes, breast changes, pubic, facial, axillary, and scalp hair changes, etc.).

SEIZURE—*see* CONVULSIONS, page 51.

SIBLING—brother or sister.

SIGMOIDOSCOPE—see Proctoscope.

SIGN—any objective evidence of a disease.

SONOGRAM—noninvasive evaluation of internal body structures using reflected ultrasound waves.

SPUTUM—mucus coughed from the respiratory tract.

STENOSIS—narrowing.

STEROIDS—potent medications (with many side effects) that tend to reduce inflammation.

STRABISMUS—walleyed, cross-eyed.

SYMPATHOMIMETIC—a medication that acts like the sympathetic nervous system (ephedrine, amphetamine). Sympathetic effects are fast heart rate and increased blood pressure.

SYMPATHOLYTIC—a medication that reduces the effects of the sympathetic nervous system (guanethedine, methyldopa).

SYMPTOM—a change in health that the person perceives and expresses.

SYNCOPE—temporary loss of consciousness.